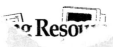

Knowledge Set

Infection Prevention & Control

Pat Ayling

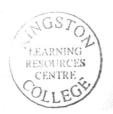

www.harcourt.co.uk

✓ Free online support
✓ Useful weblinks
✓ 24 hour online ordering

01865 888118

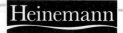

Heinemann is an imprint of Harcourt Education Limited, a company incorporated in England and Wales, having its registered office: Halley Court, Jordan Hill, Oxford OX2 8EJ. Registered company number: 3099304

www.harcourt.co.uk

Heinemann is the registered trademark of Harcourt Education Ltd

Text © Harcourt Education Ltd 2007

First published 2007

12 11 10 09 08 07
10 9 8 7 6 5 4 3 2 1

British Library Cataloguing in Publication Data is available from the British Library on request.

ISBN: 978 0 43540232 7

Typeset by TexTech International Private Ltd
Printed in the UK by Ashford Colour Press Ltd
Illustrated by Sam Thompson/Colow & Croddock and Tower Designs
Original illustrations © Harcourt Education Limited 2007
Cover design by David Poole
Cover photo: © Noelle Pollington/Flowerphotos

Websites
Please note that the examples of websites suggested in this book were up to date at the time of writing. We have made all links available on the Heinemann website at www.heinemann.co.uk/hotlinks. When you access the site, the express code is 2323P.

Contents

Introduction

Knowledge sets have been created by Skills for Care, part of the sector skills council. The idea behind each knowledge set is to provide key learning outcomes for specific areas of work within adult social care. This means that employers and training providers can use a knowledge set to provide in-house training as part of employees' continuing professional development. The advantage of using a knowledge set for the basis of training is that both employers and those who have undertaken training can be assured that a minimum standard has been reached. The knowledge sets also ensure consistency in knowledge and understanding across organisations and services.

The knowledge set for infection prevention and control is aimed at those working in social care and those hoping to do so in the future. This book has been written by Pat Ayling, who has many years' experience of nursing care in a range of settings. She now manages her own specialist health training company, is an external verifier for the awarding body, Edexcel, and an associate lecturer at Sheffield Hallam University. Using this book, in conjunction with the Skills for Care knowledge set, will:

- provide essential learning for all aspects of infection control management
- develop the skills and knowledge base of those involved in caring for vulnerable others
- support those completing NVQ and other training, providing evidence for portfolios
- support transition between different service settings in the social care sector
- ensure up-to-date and good practice.

The book is divided into the four main areas of the knowledge set:
- Cause and spread of infection
- Preventing and controlling the spread of infection
- Legislation relevant to infection prevention and control
- Roles, responsibilities and boundaries.

These sections are further broken down into manageable topics, with spreads covering one or more learning outcomes. The following features have been designed to enhance the learning experience:

Activities – completion of the suggested activities and tasks will develop understanding and skills.

Care scenarios – real-life situations allowing knowledge to be put into practice.

Look it up – pointers to recognised reference sources that allow comparison of current knowledge with accepted good practice. You may also be asked to investigate your care setting's current procedures and practices.

Reflection – explore your level of knowledge as well as your thoughts, actions and behaviours.

 Remember – key concepts and facts are highlighted and reinforced.

 Question check – test your understanding and recall of a topic.

Space has often been provided for note-taking or the completion of activities and tables, although a notebook or workbook can be used alongside this book in order to expand on certain areas.

This book not only covers the learning outcomes for those undertaking training, but also includes a section for those developing or leading training sessions. The Trainer notes provide the answers to Care scenarios, guidance on the completion of activities and also expands on the knowledge given in the four main knowledge set areas. In addition, guidance on activities within the book often includes ideas and suggestions for developing an activity and expanding on learning opportunities. Useful icons appear with each activity guidance feature, suggesting how long to spend on the activity and any materials that will be needed (e.g. pens, flip chart, OHP).

The Student log section of this book details all four main areas of the knowledge set for infection prevention and control, along with the learning outcomes. Space is provided for trainees to log their progress and record those learning outcomes they have covered. In addition, the tables can also be used to map the content of this book against NVQ courses and any other relevant training being undertaken.

Used either as part of a training package or on its own by an individual, this *Knowledge set for infection prevention and control* will prove to be an invaluable resource for those developing their career in the adult social care sector.

Acknowledgements

Harcourt would like to thank Skills for Care for giving permission to reproduce the tables of learning outcomes used in the Student Log section of this book.

The publisher and author would like to thank Jenny Chen, Education and Development Manager at The Bath Royal United Hospital, for her constructive review of this book. Thanks also to Carl Stevenson of April Park Nursing and Care Centre, Eckington, and to Cathy Wakefield at the Infection Control Unit, Rotherham District General Hospital.

We would also like to thank Professor Dinah Gould at City University, London for her invaluable advice.

Photos

Page 30 – © Photofusion/Clarissa Leahy; page 34 – (a) © iStickphoto/Oliver Sun Kim, (b) © iStickphoto/arlindo71, (c) © Steve Gschmeissner/Science Photo Library, (d) © Dr. P. Marazzi/ Science Photo Library; page 37 – © Science Photo Library/Juergen Berger; page 39 – © Science Photo Library/Kent Wood; page 45 – © Harcourt Education Ltd. Jules Selmes; page 47 – © Alamy/Jacky Chapman; page 54 – © Harcourt Education Ltd. Jules Selmes; page 63 – © Harcourt Education Ltd. Jules Selmes.

1.1 Understand the definition of infection and colonisation

Theresa McBain had read about the poor hygiene in our hospitals and care homes and so was filled with dread when her mother, Molly, was admitted with suspected colitis.

Molly however was warmly greeted, placed in an isolation room and all procedures carefully explained to her. She knew exactly why specimens were needed and what would happen to her during her stay.

What was more important was the beautifully clean room she was to stay in. She could keep all her own toiletries, had en-suite provision and a bell for 'room service', she laughed. I suspect her laughter was largely relief at the cleanliness of the hospital, the bed and the environment.

The healthcare staff from the cleaners to the assistants, the nurses and doctors were kind, considerate and always explained what they were doing and why.

'They all washed their hands thoroughly,' she said, 'so impressively clean. I am not worried any more about coming into a hospital or a care home. The standard is very high.'

'It was a pleasure to be so well cared for,' she stated after her discharge (which was soon afterwards).

micro-organism

*disease-causing micro-organisms are termed **pathogens** and mainly consist of bacteria, viruses and fungi. Infestations can also occur through parasitic organisms, which need to feed off the body to survive; examples include fleas, tapeworms and head lice. If a person or object has come into contact with a pathogen then he/she/it is said to be **contaminated***

This is how we as professional carers want all our clients to feel. It is the focus of this book to help healthcare workers understand the issues underlying potential contamination and to fully promote the prevention and control of infection.

Micro-organisms are everywhere – in dust, soil, water; on animals, pets, birds and insects. They can be found on objects such as work surfaces, dishcloths and towels. People carry them on their hands and skin and they are also found inside the body. Most are harmless and serve a useful purpose by preventing more harmful microbes from multiplying and causing disease. You need to understand about micro-organisms in order to appreciate the practices in your workplace.

The body's immune system is usually very good at fighting any pathogens that enter the body. To do this, however, the system has to be strong and healthy. Although there is no conclusive evidence, it appears to help if we:

- eat a balanced diet
- get plenty of exercise and fresh air
- sleep well
- maintain a positive attitude towards life.

People who are ill are vulnerable to infection, since their immune system will probably be weakened.

As care workers you will need to protect the individuals in your care as much as possible from the threat of infection, both **systemic** and **localised**. To do this you must be able to recognise the signs and symptoms of both types of infection. This will mean observing individuals for any warning signs of infection and understanding the nature of pathogens and how they cause illness. It is also important to be aware of the role of useful organisms that grow on the skin and in the body. These **colonise** (multiply), to protect against pathogens.

What you need to learn

- Systemic infection affects the whole body
- Localised infection is confined to a specific area
- The difference between infection and colonisation

The simplest and most effective way of preventing and controlling infection is to wash hands thoroughly and frequently, using the correct technique.

pathogen

micro-organism with the ability to cause disease

infection

the presence of micro-organisms in the body that cause illness

contamination

when something has become infected or polluted

systemic infection

infection affecting the whole body

localised infection

infection affecting a specific area of the body, for example a finger or knee

colonisation

when micro-organisms multiply in the tissues but do not cause signs or symptoms of disease

Systemic infection affects the whole body

Systemic infections have the ability to make a person feel really ill. They include measles, tuberculosis, mumps, chickenpox, whooping cough and meningitis. The sick, the elderly, babies and children are most at risk of systemic infections.

Signs and symptoms of systemic infection

The **signs** and **symptoms** of a systemic infection include:

- headache (symptom)
- high temperature (symptom – person feels hot; sign – raised thermometer reading)
- flushed (sign – red, dry skin)
- chilled (sign – shivering)
- lethargy or fatigue (sign – individual is listless, with little energy)
- vomiting (sign)
- nausea (symptom)
- general change in behaviour (sign)
- aching limbs (symptom).

Activity 1

Can you recall having a systemic infection? What did it feel like? List the signs and symptoms you experienced.

Different pathogens, different effects

The reason why a person with a systemic infection feels so ill is that, once inside the body, pathogens cause damage to body tissues. The body tissues affected vary depending on the type of pathogen present and how well the immune system reacts. Elderly people may not exhibit the classic signs and symptoms because they have weaker immune systems.

- Some pathogens attack skin cells, causing them to break down; this appears as a rash.
- Some attack the respiratory system and cause damage to the lungs (as in tuberculosis), resulting in excessive coughing and sputum production.
- Other pathogens affect brain tissue or the heart. For example, measles can progress to affect the brain, and rheumatic fever can damage heart valves, which can lead to problems in later life.

sign

what you can see about a person when he or she is unwell

symptom

what a person may complain of when he or she is unwell, for example feeling sick

- Mumps causes large swellings in the glands in the neck.
- Other infections can lead to severe blood disorders. For example, some cases of meningitis can give rise to the blood-poisoning condition septicaemia.

How systemic infection occurs

Typically, large numbers of pathogens are required to cause illness. They also need to gain entry to the body. (You can read more about the chain of infection on page 18.) The entry pathways include:

- inhalation – breathing in contaminated air
- ingestion – eating contaminated food or drinking contaminated water
- by cracks or breaks in the skin, for example an insect bite.

Pathogens can also release **toxins** – poisons that are actually the waste material or part of the bacterial cell wall. Toxins travel in the bloodstream, causing many or all of the signs and symptoms of infection. In severe cases, particularly those affecting the young, elderly and sick, these pathogens can cause collapse and even death.

toxins
poisons released from pathogenic microbes

Malaria

Malaria, although uncommon in the UK, is a potentially life-threatening illness that affects humans in tropical regions. It is caused by a parasite that lives inside the Anopheles mosquito. The illustration below shows the life cycle of the Anopheles mosquito. Note how being bitten by the mosquito results in **transmission** of the malarial parasite into a person's bloodstream, resulting in the systemic infection known as malaria.

transmission
the transfer between one victim and another

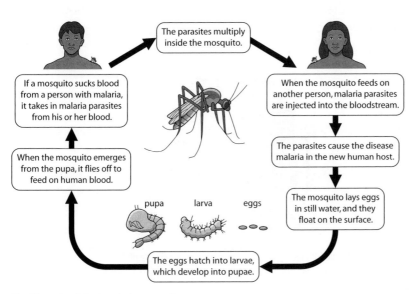

The life cycle of the Anopheles mosquito

Activity 2

Complete a table like the one below for different systemic infections.

Disease	How it is transmitted	Body part affected	Signs and symptoms of illness

Localised infection is confined to a specific area

Imagine you are bitten by a dog or an insect. The area affected will quickly become red, painful and swollen. Occasionally there will be a discharge of pus. If there are no further symptoms in other areas of your body, this is known as a localised infection. But should the infection spread or get into the bloodstream, it becomes a systemic infection.

Types of localised infection

Abscess

An abscess, or boil, is typically a very inflamed area where the skin has been broken, allowing pathogens to enter and multiply. Typical signs include redness, swelling, a collection of pus (a yellow/white discharge) and pain. These signs are called the **inflammatory response**. Squeezing a spot or boil with dirty fingers will introduce pathogens to the area. A root abscess occurs when pathogens enter a decayed tooth and spread to the root.

inflammatory response

the body's reaction to infection whereby white blood cell activity and antibodies at the site of infection have caused redness, swelling and the collection of pus (dead white cells)

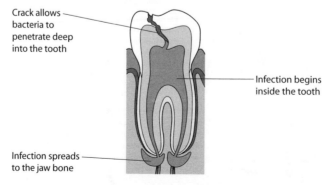

Crack allows bacteria to penetrate deep into the tooth

Infection begins inside the tooth

Infection spreads to the jaw bone

An abscess is an example of a localised infection that is extremely painful

Bites and stings

When the skin's surface is broken by an animal bite or sting, it becomes possible for pathogens the animal is carrying to enter the body. Pathogens may enter in the form of venom, or may be present in the animal's saliva.

Without treatment the infection may spread along a tract, for example a bite on the lower arm may result in an inflammatory response up to the elbow over a short period of time. Localised infections can progress to become systemic, so it is essential to seek medical attention immediately if you notice this happening.

Cuts and grazes

Pathogens that live in the soil can get into wounds that happen outdoors or while using garden tools. Tetanus is one example of a serious disease caused by pathogens living in the soil entering the body, usually through deep penetrating wounds. The pathogens live in contaminated manure and can cause systemic problems such as muscle spasms and kidney failure.

A localised infection can occur if you persistently scratch itchy or irritated skin, thereby breaking the skin's surface. Sometimes glands near the site of a localised infection become swollen. For example, if you have a cut on your finger, the glands in your armpit may become enlarged. This is because the glands release huge numbers of white blood cells to fight the infection.

Infections are always caused by pathogens. These micro-organisms have different properties and can damage body tissues in different ways. Pathogens include bacteria, viruses, fungi (in the form of moulds or yeasts) and parasites.

Care scenario: Harry

Harry is an 85-year-old man who has cut his finger with his penknife. His finger is now red, swollen and painful.

1. What do you think has happened?
2. Besides a cut, what else may cause a localised inflammatory response?

Activity 3

1. List three signs of infection that you might notice in an individual.

2. List three complaints that may indicate that an individual is suffering from infection.

The difference between infection and colonisation

Some strains of micro-organisms will divide and multiply in the human body without causing disease (for example, types of specific bacteria such as *Clostridium difficile*, see page 25). A person is said to be 'colonised' by that organism; 30–40 per cent of people are colonised by *Staphylococcus aureas*, which lives on the skin, in the nasal passages, groin area and armpits. This causes no problems until that person sustains an open wound or undergoes a surgical operation. At that point the organism becomes a threat and could produce enzymes or toxins (poisons) that cause tissue damage. It can also be spread to others.

These colonies normally protect the body from pathogenic bacteria by overwhelming them when they enter body tissue, hence they are sometimes referred to as healthy bacteria. *E. coli* is another organism that lives happily in the gut causing no harm. If, however, a person's immune system is weak or compromised, infection can occur by the production of enzymes damaging healthy cells.

Infection occurs when pathogens enter the body and multiply in tissue, causing the signs and indications of disease. This can occur when a person colonised by a particular type of pathogen passes them to others. Transmission may be via:

- air, e.g. coughing and sneezing
- blood, e.g. an injection with a contaminated needle
- body fluids, e.g. semen during unprotected sex
- direct contact, e.g. touching with contaminated hands.

The colonised person is termed a **carrier**. Carriers can be convalescent (recovering from illness) or healthy individuals. With some bacterial infections we need to check for the presence of responsible pathogens in the faeces following an illness. This is

carrier

a person infected with a pathogen that remains in the body but causes no signs of illness

Activity 4: De-colonisation

Complete a table like the one below to say how you as a healthcare worker can prevent pathogens colonising and causing infections.

Pathogenic organisms can colonise via...	I can help to stop this by...
Coughing and sneezing	
Blood and body fluids	
Direct contact	
Ingestion	

important for those working with sick individuals or handling food. Faeces must be clear of contamination to eliminate the risk of **cross-infection**. The risk of cross-infection from a carrier is much greater for individuals whose ability to fight disease is lowered. For example, a person may be a carrier of MRSA (see page 24) and pass this on to vulnerable others who become infected and very ill.

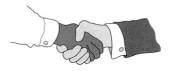

Carrier A   Person B

Carrier A shakes hands with non-carrier Person B

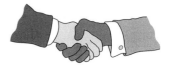

Carrier B   Person C

B, now a carrier, contaminates Person C

Carriers carry pathogens without showing signs of illness. They are capable of transmitting pathogens to others who then become ill

Care scenario: Laura

Laura is a care assistant who has just returned from a holiday in the Far East, where she suffered from diarrhoea and vomiting. She has recovered and is back at work today.

1. What do you think may have caused Laura's diarrhoea and vomiting?
2. Explain the potential health risk to the individuals in Laura's care.
3. Why do you think Laura is a potential threat?

cross-infection

process by which micro-organisms on one object or person transfer to another object or person (e.g. dishcloth to food)

Activity 5

Create a mind-map like the one below for each of the following key terms, to help build your knowledge:

- localised infections
- systemic infections
- colonisation.

Localised infections

For each mind-map, add as much detail as you can and try to use all of the key words (in **bold**) introduced in this section.

1. Define infection.
2. What is the difference between localised and systemic infection?
3. Where are pathogens found?
4. What is the difference between a sign and a symptom of infection?
5. What do you understand by colonisation?
6. What does contamination mean?
7. List four possible signs and symptoms in a person suffering from a systemic infection.
8. Why are babies, young children, the elderly and the sick especially prone to infections?

It is important to understand that some micro-organisms provide protection for the body and do it no harm. These are called **normal floras**. Understanding how micro-organisms can be useful in the body helps with infection control. The body is good at maintaining a balance of pathogens and ensuring that those which attack healthy tissues are speedily removed from the body; in the case of food poisoning, for example, this is by vomiting and/or diarrhoea.

normal floras

helpful non-pathogenic organisms

This section explores:

- the role of normal floras and when they might become troublesome
- the body's other defences against harmful micro-organisms
- how microbes, once established in the body, can cause damage to other people.

In the workplace you will need to know how normal floras help to protect individuals from disease, how pathogens cause disease, and how to maintain awareness of infection control by consistently breaking the chain of infection.

What you will need to learn

- How non-pathogenic organisms within the body (often called normal floras) and body mechanisms help fight disease
- How pathogens cause disease
- The chain of infection

How non-pathogenic organisms within the body (often called normal floras) and body mechanisms help fight disease

The role of normal floras within the body

These helpful micro-organisms are sometimes called resident micro-organisms. Their presence is very important in preventing pathogens from colonising the skin or the intestines, for example. This is because the pathogens prefer to grow where there are no other micro-organisms to compete with. The huge numbers of normal floras therefore discourage any pathogens from multiplying further, and in this way help the human body stay healthy and fight infection.

Another role of normal floras is to aid digestion. They live in the large intestine in great numbers, which protects against pathogens (see above). Resident floras also produce vitamin K, which plays an important role in blood clotting.

Saprophytes are normal floras found in the body and on the skin; they eat dead cells and pathogens. Outside the gut, these micro-organisms are essential in nature's recycling process, breaking down dead plant and animal matter to provide nutrients for plant and animal feed.

Normal floras are also used in the production of:

- antibiotics, for example streptomycin for tuberculosis
- some foodstuffs, for example cheese and yoghurt
- insulin, which is essential to controlling blood sugar levels in diabetics.

Other micro-organisms that do not harm the body are some fungi:

- penicillium is a type of mould used as the antibiotic penicillin
- many mushrooms are safe for eating, however some varieties are poisonous
- yeasts are used in bread and beer, and in the formation of alcohol.

When normal floras may become troublesome

Problems can arise if normal floras get into parts of the body where they are not normally found, for example floras from the gut getting into the urethra or vagina. Here, the body does not recognise the micro-organisms as being normally in that area and so colonisation can cause problems, such as irritation and infection. This can also happen following over-use of antibiotics, which may strip the normal flora along with the pathogenic bacteria.

Body mechanisms to fight infection

To fight off infections efficiently, the body needs to be in a healthy condition. This means having a high level of **immunity**, which is achieved by eating a balanced, nutritious diet and following a healthy lifestyle (see also pages 52–3). Sometimes, however, an individual's immunity is lowered and his or her resistance to infection is poor. People needing care are in this category. The very young, the elderly and those who are unwell can have periods of lower immunity, particularly during stressful periods.

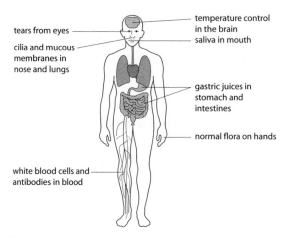

The body's defences against infection

temperature control in the brain
saliva in mouth
tears from eyes
cilia and mucous membranes in nose and lungs
gastric juices in stomach and intestines
normal flora on hands
white blood cells and antibodies in blood

immunity

the body's ability to ward off infection. This can be natural, as in the case of antibodies fighting antigens, or artificial, for example the result of immunisation or vaccination

Stress appears to lower immunity. We don't really know why, but a positive attitude seems to help people stay healthy. It is important to look after yourself and others with this in mind. Encouraging a positive outlook and time to relax rather than a negative focus on illness may actually speed up recovery from infection.

Skin

Skin consists of two layers:

- The epidermis is the skin's tough outer layer which serves as a physical barrier against infection. It is also slightly acidic. This creates a natural antiseptic effect that helps to slow the spread of bacteria on the skin (see also pages 44–5).

- The dermis is the skin's inner layer. It consists of loose jelly-like connective tissue. Here, **secretions** made by glands protect the skin from cracking, which would allow pathogens to enter.

secretion

substance produced by the cells of the body, for example tears or mucus

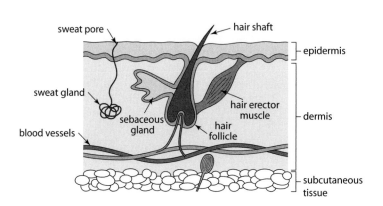

sweat pore
hair shaft
epidermis
sweat gland
hair erector muscle
sebaceous gland
hair follicle
blood vessels
dermis
subcutaneous tissue

The skin on the hands is home to huge numbers of resident floras, which help to deter any pathogens (see also pages 4–5). You can scrub your hands for a long time but you would not be able to remove their natural floras. However, **transient floras**, for example salmonella found on raw meat, can remain on the hands for quite a while, so the risk of cross-infection is high.

transient floras

organisms easily acquired on the hands through touch and transferable to another person or surface

Care scenario: Dennis

Dennis works in the staff canteen of the local hospital. The canteen is busy, with long queues of people waiting to be served. Dennis has been called from the kitchen area, where he has been preparing raw meat, to help with serving meals. He washes his hands with soap on the way out, but does not wash them very thoroughly because he is in a rush to serve people.

1. What may be the consequences of Dennis not washing his hands properly for the people he serves food to?
2. What could the consequences for the hospital be if there was an outbreak of food poisoning in the canteen?

Establishments serving food, such as hotels, shops and restaurants, as well as hospitals, nursing homes and residential homes, are fined a lot of money for causing outbreaks of food poisoning. This is a crime and is one reason why strict policies on food hygiene are vital. How would you feel if you were the cause of someone suffering an infection because you did not wash your hands properly or follow the correct hygiene procedures? (Proper hand-washing is discussed on pages 44–45.)

Using the Internet or reference books, research the laws that deal with food poisoning. (You may also want to refer to pages 69–70.)

Mucous membranes

Secretions from mucous membranes in the nose and lining of the lungs help to trap pathogens, which are then sneezed, coughed or blown out of the body.

Tears

Without tears, the eyes would be dry and vulnerable to infection. Tears include an antibacterial substance called lysozyme. They also move any dust and particles that have entered the eye to the inner corner of the eye, where they are easily removed.

Saliva

Saliva has anti-bacterial properties. As food is chewed, it helps to break down harmful particles, killing off potential pathogens before they are swallowed.

Cilia

Cilia are tiny hair-like projections that help to remove harmful pathogens from the body by wafting them towards the exterior. They are found in the lining of the lungs and the nasal passages.

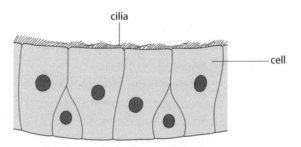

Cilia in the nasal passages

White blood cells

White blood cells increase their number in the body when they recognise foreign material – that is, when an **antigen** has entered the body. Deceased white blood cells appear as pus at the site of a localised infection. Blood clotting seals wounds, stopping any further pathogens from entering.

Some white blood cells are called macrophages and their job is to swallow antigens.

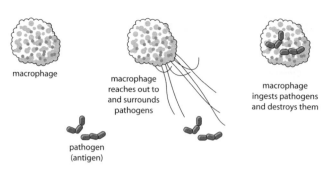

macrophage

macrophage reaches out to and surrounds pathogens

macrophage ingests pathogens and destroys them

pathogen (antigen)

How a macrophage eats up and destroys an antigen

Antibodies

Antibodies are formed from special memory cells in the body. They recognise antigens from previous infections and seek them out and stick to them, enabling the macrophages to engulf the antigens. This is why you will only catch chickenpox once in your lifetime, even if you come into contact with this **contagious** disease more than once: your memory cells will recognise the antigen (chickenpox virus) and call in the antibodies to fight it off.

New antigens challenge the body to produce different antibodies and this can take some time, especially if the immune system is weakened. Antibodies are also created by the **inoculation** of tiny amounts of antigens. You may remember some of the inoculations you were given as a child. You may also have been inoculated against diseases such as yellow fever, before travelling abroad. Inoculations of this kind will be given several weeks before you travel, to allow your body time to produce efficient antibodies.

Temperature control

When pathogens enter the body, there is often a rise in body temperature that may be the body's attempt to reduce the number of pathogenic micro-organisms by preventing growth. However it is useful to remember that elderly people may suffer infections but show no rise in temperature. The body's ability to fight infection is lessened in this group of people.

contagious

(infection) easily spread from one person to another

inoculation

injecting an artificially made vaccine to protect the body against pathogens that cause disease. The terms 'inoculation' and 'immunisation' are often used interchangeably

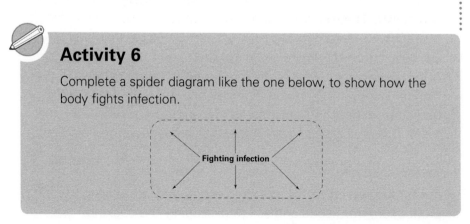

Activity 6

Complete a spider diagram like the one below, to show how the body fights infection.

Fighting infection

How do pathogenic organisms cause disease?

The right conditions for growth

Pathogens are invisible to the naked eye but are everywhere. They are living organisms and need a suitable environment in which to grow. The ideal conditions in which they thrive are described below.

Temperature

The ideal temperature is known as ambient or room temperature (approximately 20–45 degrees Celsius). Pathogens rarely survive above 85 degrees Celsius or below 4 degrees Celsius. The ideal temperature for the growth of human pathogens is the body temperature, i.e. 37 degrees Celsius.

Moisture

Damp favours the growth of pathogenic micro-organisms. Some, for example cholera, can grow in water, but most do not. A few yeasts, moulds and fungi grow in dry conditions.

pH balance

Most pathogens prefer **pH** neutral or alkaline environments, generally not liking acidic conditions. One exception is *Staphylococcus aureas*, which grows well in low-pH or acidic conditions.

Oxygen

Most pathogens grow successfully in oxygen, though some can survive with no oxygen; these are called anaerobic.

Time

Pathogens need time to divide and carry on multiplying. Some pathogens will multiply very quickly, while others do so more slowly.

Transient floras

Normal floras may pass from their 'normal' area to one that is alien to them, causing irritations and possibly infections. An example of this is bacteria from the anus entering the urethra (tube to the bladder which is quite short in females) if the female has wiped herself from back to front instead of front to back after using the toilet. This may lead to cystitis (bacterial infection of the bladder).

In the food chain

Contamination by pathogens can occur at any stage of food production, from seed and soil to packaging and cooking.

pH (percentage of hydrogen ions)

The pH scale ranges from 0 (strongly acidic) to 14.0 (strongly alkaline). A pH of 7.0 is neutral (neither acidic or alkaline)

Most pathogens thrive in moist, warm conditions (the human body temperature of 37 degrees Celsius is ideal) with plenty of oxygen and nutrients. They prefer a pH neutral environment, generally not liking acidic conditions, and they need time to multiply.

- Where animals are involved for meat production, the carcass (dead body of the animal) may become contaminated through inadequate storage temperatures (pathogens like warmth). Poor hygiene during butchering may also contribute.

- A few pathogens can survive freezing and dark conditions, for example in soil. When conditions become favourable again – that is, when warmth and oxygen are present – they start to multiply once again. A few types of bacteria have a coating that protects them in harsh conditions such as heat and freezing. This coating is termed a **spore**, and has the property of germinating and multiplying once conditions become favourable again, i.e. when warmth, moisture and food are available.

- Organisms can be transferred in an indirect way, for example from raw meat to a ready-to-eat food such as a sandwich (this is an example of cross-infection or cross-contamination).

- Cooking at too low a temperature or for too short a time will result in pathogens still being present in food and able to carry on multiplying.

- Not stirring hot food sufficiently to avoid 'cool spots'.

- The core temperature of cooked meat should be checked with a probe (disinfected after use) which should read a minimum of 75 degrees Celsius for 3 minutes.

- Re-heating should ensure this **minimum** temperature and should only happen once.

> **spores**
>
> *protective coatings on some bacteria that make them hard to destroy even at very high or low temperatures. If conditions become favourable, the spores germinate to enable the bacteria to multiply*

Transient in water

Pathogens can survive in water so can be taken into the body via drinking water or contaminated seafood. The UK has hygiene controls to prevent this, but where these do not exist it is likely that water will be polluted and cause illness. Legionnaires' disease (see also page 24) is caused by contaminated water systems and there are occasional outbreaks in the UK.

People to people; insects to animals; animals to people

- Insects can bite animals and people and introduce pathogens into the body. These are then transported into the bloodstream (see also the example of malaria on page 5).

- Animals can pass on pathogens via their blood, saliva, urine or faeces. If pets are handled and the hands become contaminated, the pathogens will live on the hands until they are removed by washing or move on to food or another person.

- Pathogens can be transferred from person to person via sexual contact (through semen and vaginal secretions).

Transient in dust and air

Invisible but potentially harmful organisms can be breathed in. Environments such as continuously circulating air in aeroplanes or in cooling systems may contain pathogens. Coughing and sneezing release tiny droplets of infected mucus into the air; this transports pathogens to others resulting in, for example, colds or influenza.

Transient on objects

If objects such as dishcloths, tea towels and wash towels become contaminated, the organisms can survive until they are transported on to something else, for example food or another person. Objects that have the potential to pass transient floras on to others are called **fomites**.

fomite

an item or piece of equipment, for example towels, face cloths, tables, chairs, books, toys, that can pass on a disease from an infected person to others

Activity 7

1. List the possible behaviours or actions that may aid the movement of transient pathogens.

2. List the objects that might easily become infected by transient pathogens.

The chain of infection

The different stages by which transient floras succeed in causing infection are termed the chain of infection. The chain of infection is used to illustrate how pathogens move from one host to the next. In order to prevent infection, you need to break this chain.

Pathogens

The chain begins with the pathogens (bacteria, viruses or fungi).

Environment

The second link of the chain is the environment. Factors that determine environmental conditions for growth are:

- food, or nutrients
- moisture
- temperature
- oxygen
- pH (neutral, alkaline or acidic environment)
- time to multiply.

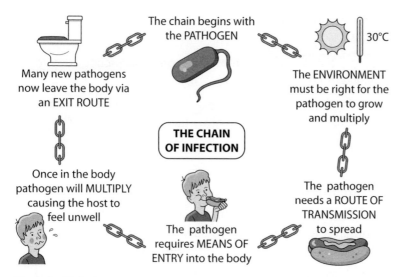

The chain of infection

Most pathogens flourish in moist, warm conditions with plenty of oxygen and nutrients (see also page 36). Damp food or a humid atmosphere provide the perfect conditions for growth. However, there are exceptions:

- Some micro-organisms prefer hot environments; these are called thermophilics but they rarely cause human infections.

- Some micro-organisms prefer cold, even freezing temperatures. This is one reason why cook–chill foods come with a 'use before' date on the package.

- Anaerobic bacteria can survive when there is no oxygen. These are often found in the soil but can get into the food chain.

- Some bacteria produce spores (see page 17) that can survive unfavourable conditions. When conditions become favourable again, the spores produce pathogenic micro-organisms which multiply rapidly. Spores can exist in freezing conditions in soil or water for months, even years. They can also survive for long periods on objects such as those contained in a sluice! Examples of spore-producing bacteria are *Clostridium botulinum* (which causes severe food poisoning and can be isolated in soil), and *Clostridium difficile* (which can cause severe diarrhoea and is prevalent in healthcare settings as an airborne pathogen).

- To eradicate *Clostridium botulinum* from the food industry, the preservation method of canning involves exposure to extremely high heat for a certain period of time. Spore-producing bacteria are kept at bay by avoiding the danger zone of temperatures between 5 and 63 degrees Celsius.

Activity 8

1. Why is it important to wash root vegetables properly before eating them?

2. When food is stored in a fridge or freezer, why does it still have the potential to grow transient pathogens?

Route of transmission

The third link in the chain of infection is the route that the organism requires to spread. As we saw on page 17–18, transmission may be via the following methods:

- Ingestion of contaminated food or water. For example, eating undercooked poultry or minced beef or sausages can result in a food-borne illness, as can eating a sandwich that has been contaminated by the preparer's unwashed hands.

- Inhalation of contaminated air. This can happen in viral infections when particles from faeces or vomit become airborne.

- Contamination through a break in the skin, for example a cut, or via body fluids.

- Direct contamination by touch, e.g. by the hands.

The route by which a pathogen enters the body is known as the **portal of entry**.

portal of entry

how a pathogen enters the body

Enter and multiply

Once in a new environment where conditions are favourable, transient pathogens will start to multiply by dividing in two. This is called **binary fission** and can happen quickly or slowly, depending on the organism type. The process continues until there are huge numbers of microbes. If the pathogens have invaded a human host, it is at this stage that the signs and symptoms of infectious illness (see page 4) become apparent.

binary fission

process by which a single-celled organism splits into two cells of roughly equal size

It can take as little as 15–20 minutes for a bacterium to divide. Thus billions may be present in just 24 hours.

Exit routes

Pathogens will start to die if environmental conditions become unfavourable. However, if **excreted** from their host via faeces, saliva or mucus, they can hitch a ride to another host via, for example, hands, food or inanimate objects known as fomites (see also page 18).

Another example is a shared toy which contains pathogens that left the body via nasal discharge. The means by which a pathogen exits the body is known as the **portal of exit**.

excrete

to get rid of waste from the body

portal of exit

how a pathogen leaves the body

Activity 9

1. What everyday actions do you perform to break the chain of infection?

2. Give examples of unacceptable practice for each link in the chain of infection.

Activity 10

For each of the terms below, write all the words you can think of associated with it. Try to add some meanings. You could do this by drawing a mind-map around each word. Some words will have been mentioned earlier in the book, but only look back if you get stuck.

- normal flora
- portal of entry
- portal of exit
- transmission
- pathogen growth conditions
- body mechanisms to fight infection
- examples of contaminated objects.

1. Describe normal flora.

2. Describe how transient pathogens can enter the body.

3. List three body mechanisms that give protection from pathogens.

4. Give an example of how a care worker can contaminate a wound.

5. Why might the body take a long time to produce antibodies?

6. Explain how immunisation programmes protect people from pathogens.

7. What is contamination?

8. List five requirements for the successful growth of pathogens.

9. What is a spore?

Pathogenic micro-organisms can be anywhere, and we are particularly at risk from virulent types. However we can play an important role in preventing disease if in our role as healthcare workers we always practise excellent hygiene controls. If people are vulnerable, for example because of illness or living in conditions of poverty, then their body is weakened and they are more likely to become ill with infections caused by pathogenic micro-organisms such as bacteria and viruses. Fungal infections commonly affect the skin, and parasites are tiny living creatures that are transmitted to others by physical contact, for example head lice or scabies. It is important to know that perfectly clean people can be the victims of scabies and lice.

What you will need to learn

- Bacteria – their structure and properties, and examples of diseases they cause
- Viruses – their structure and properties, and examples of diseases they cause
- Fungi – their structure and properties, and the conditions they cause
- Parasites – the different types and how they affect the human body

Bacteria

The structure and properties of bacteria

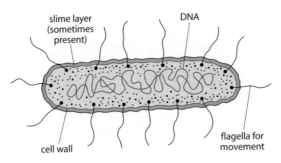

The structure of a typical bacterium

The structure and properties of bacteria enable them to survive and multiply. Nutrients are absorbed through the cell wall and waste products are excreted in the same way. The waste products of bacteria are sometimes referred to as toxins or poisons, and it is these that cause unpleasant effects in the body, such as vomiting and diarrhoea.

A bacterium divides into two and copies itself within a short space of time (20–30 minutes in ideal conditions) by a process called *binary fission* (see also page 20). When available nutrients are used up, the bacteria begin to die off or are excreted from the body and continue to survive in another environment, for example in faeces.

Some facts about bacteria

- A single bacterium is about one-thousandth of a millimetre long.
- Flagella are very fine hair-like structures that help bacteria to move through water and body tissues.
- Bacteria are usually divided into three different types: cocci, bacilli and spirochetes.
- These are different shapes of bacteria that can be seen under a microscope. Each type produces different effects in the body.
- Some bacteria are beneficial in that they break down dead animal and vegetable matter, so aiding the recycling of nutrients for the food chain.

Large numbers of bacteria together with the best conditions for their growth are needed to cause illness.

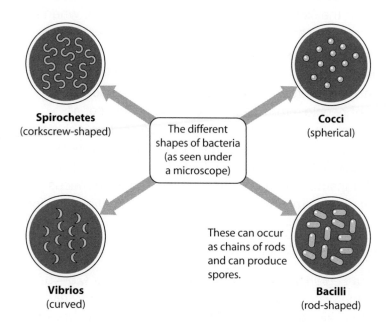

Spirochetes (corkscrew-shaped)

Cocci (spherical)

The different shapes of bacteria (as seen under a microscope)

Vibrios (curved)

These can occur as chains of rods and can produce spores.

Bacilli (rod-shaped)

The most alarming property of bacteria is their ability to mutate (to change shape or metabolic activity). This has been highlighted in recent years with the arrival of MRSA (see page 24) and other bacteria that appear to be resistant to treatment with antibiotics. The resulting campaign in many hospitals and care homes is designed to promote safe hygiene practices to effectively manage infection control. (You will look at these strategies in more detail in Unit 2.1.)

Examples of diseases caused by pathogenic bacteria

MRSA (*methicillin resistant Staphylococcus aureas*)

This organism is proving extremely difficult to manage in hospitals and care homes. Many individuals have caught it while in hospital and it has been difficult to treat them with antibiotics. Medical personnel have concluded that MRSA bacteria have mutated in order to survive antibiotic treatment. The infection has commonly affected individuals with open wounds, for example after surgery, and is also associated with skin infections.

It is estimated that approximately 40 per cent of people are carriers of *Staphylococcus aureas*, which is present on the hands, in the throat and the nasal passages.

Prevention calls for everyone, especially healthcare workers, to be mindful of good hygiene. Once *Staphylococcus aureas* has been isolated in a urine or sputum specimen, some doctors may prescribe nasal cream or drops to help combat its presence.

The correct hand-washing procedure is described on pages 44–45.

Tuberculosis (TB)

This condition mainly affects the lungs and is caused by a bacterium called *Mycobacterium tuberculosis*. Those infected will not necessarily develop the disease – individuals with a healthy immune system will be healthy 'carriers' and will experience no symptoms. However, TB bacteria can lie dormant for many years, and in a small number of cases may be reactivated to cause the full-blown disease, usually because the immune system is weakened. TB is contagious only when the signs and symptoms are present, i.e. when a person is spreading the bacteria by coughing and sneezing (airborne transmission).

The TB skin test (mantoux) can identify people who have had the infection in the past. A positive result will indicate a degree of natural immunity; a negative result indicates increased susceptibility and highlights a need for the BCG inoculation. This would offer some protection for a large number of people. From September 2005, instead of all school children receiving inoculation, only those considered high risk do so. This includes anyone living in overcrowded conditions or with parents or grandparents who were born in countries where TB is prevalent whose TB causes sticky infected mucus and spasms of coughing, which are the cause of transmission. It is diagnosed by examining mucus coughed up from the lungs (sputum) under a microscope. It is treated with antibiotics, for example streptomycin.

Legionnaires' disease

This disease is caused by the bacteria *Legionella*, which multiply in warm water (25–45 degrees Celsius), particularly where the water or evaporative air is stagnant (not freely moving). *Legionella* is therefore found in air-conditioning systems and spread via showers and cooling systems. Rarely, people from the UK may catch the disease while on holiday.

The symptoms of Legionnaires' disease are headaches, tiredness, coughing and a high temperature. Chest x-rays may show pneumonia (respiratory disease). It frequently occurs in people over the age of 50 and in those with a weakened immune system. Treatment is by antibiotics. The disease cannot be spread from person to person.

Clostridium difficile

This bacterium is an increasing hazard in healthcare, in fact more so than the well publicised MRSA. It is an anaerobic bacterium, which means it can survive and multiply without the need for oxygen. As the large bowel contains very little oxygen, it thrives there and a diagnosis is made based on the presence of the organism in the faeces.

Over-use of antibiotics can disturb the healthy bacteria that colonise the bowel, giving rise to the release of the toxins responsible for diarrhoea. To further compound the problem, spores released in diarrhoea can easily contaminate surfaces such as toilets, skin and bed linen. They can also become airborne, for example during bed-making. Contamination of the hands is therefore very likely and they become a strong vehicle for the spread of the bacteria. Thorough and regular cleaning is paramount in the control of this hazardous pathogen. The following are most susceptible to infection:

- the immune-compromised (people who are sick or have a chronic condition that has weakened their immune system)
- people who have been treated with broad-spectrum antibiotics (antibiotics that can treat a wide range of diseases)
- the elderly
- people having bowel surgery or needing regular enemas.

It is important to be constantly aware of good hygiene practice in the quest to limit the hazards of this pathogen. Thorough cleaning of sluices, surfaces and bed areas, including careful changing and disposing of linen, is paramount. Patients infected with *Clostridium difficile* should have their own room, toilet facilities and toiletries. Staff, patients and visitors are strongly advised to wash hands thoroughly with liquid soap and water, followed by an alcohol rub.

Food-poisoning bacteria

These can be classified into causes by infective agents (e.g. bacteria, viruses and parasites) and toxic agents (e.g. poisonous mushrooms, pesticides or improper preparation of foodstuffs such as red kidney beans, which must be boiled for about 30 minutes and simmered until natural poisons have been eradicated).

Campylobacter infections

These bacteria, the most common cause of food poisoning, give rise to the infection Campylobacteriosis, which causes diarrhoea (which may be bloody), cramping, abdominal pain and fever within 2–5 days of exposure to the pathogen. It is a very common sporadic infection that can last for up to one week.

Most *Campylobacter* infections in humans are caused by the spiral-shaped *Campylobacter jejuni*. Most cases are associated with handling raw poultry or eating undercooked poultry (*Campylobacter* bacteria are present in large numbers of chickens). They can be acquired from drinking unpasteurised milk or contaminated water. Recovery may not require any treatment other than replacement of lost fluids, however in some cases antibiotics are prescribed.

Prevention consists of good hygiene in the kitchen and the avoidance of cross-contamination during the preparation of raw chicken. It is also crucial to cook the chicken to temperatures of 77–80 degrees Celsius and until juices run clear. Remember that chicken should be re-heated to these high temperatures only once and no more.

Salmonella

The second most common culprit, *Salmonella* may be found in unpasteurised milk, raw meat and poultry. The vehicles for the contaminant may therefore be certain cheeses made with unpasteurised milk, mayonnaise, sauces and salad dressings. *Salmonella* can also be transmitted by animals and household pets. The **incubation** period is usually 12–36 hours; signs and symptoms include severe abdominal pain, diarrhoea, vomiting and fever. Prevention consists of careful preparation of raw meat to avoid cross-contamination.

Staphylococcus aureas (toxin in food)

Referred to earlier as the organism implicated in cases of MRSA, where it can be identified in wounds, this toxin can multiply in cooked meat and meat products, eggs and salad produce, dairy products and some dried foods. As the toxin grows on food before it is eaten, the incubation period is short: often only 1–7 hours. Symptoms include abdominal cramps, nausea, vomiting and sometimes diarrhoea. Good personal hygiene is needed to avoid this type of food poisoning, especially hand-hygiene. Food handling while coughing and sneezing should definitely be avoided, as this pathogen is found in the nose, throat and on skin. Any cuts should be covered by blue waterproof dressings if handling food.

> **incubation**
>
> *the time taken for a pathogen or its toxins to cause the signs and symptoms of disease*

Activity 11

Think about it:

Clostridium difficile has been identified in the faecal specimen of Mrs Maloney in the care home where you are working. Today she is in your care. Mrs Maloney has an indwelling catheter and has been gently mobilising for a week, taking herself to the toilet and bathroom. What special precautions will you take on your shift today and what advice will you give Mrs Maloney and her visitors?

Tetanus

Tetanus is caused by the bacterium *Clostridium tetani* which is found in soil, commonly in animal dung and manure. These bacteria can also live in street dust and inside buildings. They give off spores that can lie dormant for years and then produce pathogenic microbes when the right conditions for growth are present.

The disease can arise from a minor injury, such as a prick from a contaminated rose thorn; however usually the injury is deep and penetrating, allowing this pathogen that does not tolerate oxygen to multiply. The toxin produced by the bacteria is highly poisonous and affects the nervous system, causing muscle rigidity, particularly of the jaw (hence the common name 'lockjaw'). This causes difficulty in swallowing and muscular paralysis. The treatment is hospitalisation and large doses of antibiotics.

Bacterial tonsillitis

Streptococcus is the most common cause of tonsillitis. Diagnosis is based on extreme soreness of the throat and swollen glands in the neck. The face may be red and flushed. It is possible that the tonsillitis is caused by a virus, in which case these symptoms would be accompanied by influenza-type signs and symptoms. A streptococcal bacterium responds well to antibiotics. Complications are rare but may lead to an abscess (quinsy).

Bacterial meningitis

Caused by close prolonged contact with a contaminated person, this condition develops rapidly. It causes severe headache, neck stiffness, nausea, vomiting and light intolerance. Victims must receive antibiotics as soon as possible to avoid the complications of septicaemia, which is apparent by the appearance of a rash not suppressed by passing a glass over the skin. The rash is caused by small haemorrhagic bleeds into the tissues of the body. Early warning signs are said to be a very high temperature but with cold hands and feet.

E. Coli (*Escherichia coli*)

Several types of these bacteria colonise the human intestine.

E. Coli 0157

This organism is commonly found in cattle and poultry; however contamination has been discovered in unpasteurised apple juice, hamburger meat, radish sprouts, lettuce, potatoes and other food sources. It is also found in water contaminated with faecal deposits. Human-to-human transmission via faecal matter has been identified in care homes.

Watery diarrhoea follows an incubation period of three to four days on average. This can quickly progress to bloody diarrhoea and gastro-intestinal symptoms of nausea and vomiting. The bacteria can produce verotoxin, which can damage small blood vessels, leading to kidney failure. Isolation of the person is essential and specimens should be taken

Activity 12

Complete a table like the one below for the bacterial infections in this section; then research at least two other bacterial diseases and add this information to the table. In the Complications column, you should write the most severe consequences of each infection.

Disease	Transmission method	Symptoms	Complications

to identify the responsible strain. Other strains can cause infections in wounds, the urinary tract and the abdominal cavity, the latter causing peritonitis. Immune-compromised patients and patients being nursed on ventilators are particularly vulnerable. Treatment depends on the strain.

Prevention involves thorough and careful preparation of all meat products if you are a food handler and scrupulous hygiene at all times when you are caring for people in community settings.

Viruses

The structure and properties of viruses

Viruses are much smaller than bacteria and can only be seen with a powerful electron microscope. Whereas bacteria need to multiply until there are significant numbers to cause disease, a virus has to enter a living 'host' cell. By releasing its DNA (deoxyribonucleic acid) or its RNA (ribonucleic acid) it changes the genetic coding of that host cell. (DNA and RNA are types of genetic material.) By a process known as uncoating, the viral coding separates from the host cell and is replicated in other cells. The host cell eventually dies and the new virus is released to find more host cells.

A virus has no metabolic activity as bacteria do and therefore does not produce waste. Antibiotics work by stopping metabolic activity, therefore they are of no use against viral infections. It has been difficult to develop drugs to kill viruses. Some antiviral drugs, however, can block the steps in the process by which viruses reproduce.

A virus can enter the body by the same routes as bacteria (see pages 5 and 20). Person-to-person spread is common.

Examples of diseases caused by viruses

HIV

The human immunodeficiency virus (HIV) causes the disease AIDS (acquired immune deficiency syndrome). In this condition, the virus kills off a special group of white blood cells (the T-helper cells) of the immune system. These cells are the ones called in to fight infection, so people with AIDS become unable to fight off infection (immuno-suppressed).

After initial contact with the virus, individuals may experience mild flu-like symptoms lasting a few days. Thereafter, the virus works silently in the body, multiplying and destroying immune cells. It may be several years before the symptoms of AIDS (the most advanced stage of HIV infection) develop. Symptoms include repeated infections, tumours, muscle wastage and lung disease.

DNA and **RNA**

deoxyribonucleic acid and ribonucleic acid provide the genetic blueprint for the physical characteristics of all living organisms

metabolism

the building up and breaking down of chemical compounds, using up and releasing energy

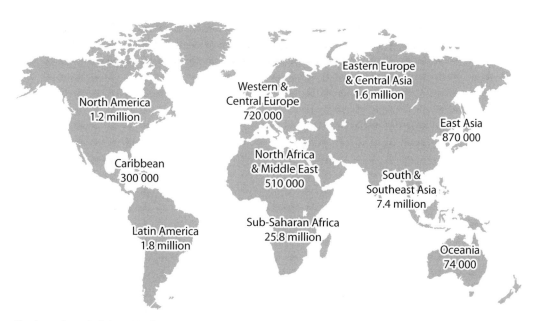

Numbers of people living with HIV infection in 2005 (Source: World Health Organization)

There are improved antiviral drugs now available to minimise the effects of AIDS.

According to the World Health Organisation (WHO), 3.1 million people died from HIV/AIDS-related causes in 2005. In that same year, the number of people estimated to be infected with the virus stood at 40 million.

Measles

Measles is transmitted via tiny airborne droplets of contaminated mucus and is highly contagious. The virus multiplies in the cells of the throat and lung passages. Symptoms include a raised temperature, coughing, vomiting and diarrhoea. Inside the mouth little white spots appear (called Koplik's spots). As the illness progresses a dusky red rash of slightly raised spots appears on the face and spreads to the neck and body. Complications include laryngitis, bronchitis and encephalitis (inflammation of the brain), which is life-threatening. Fortunately, since the introduction of the

Care scenario: MMR immunisation

Sarah is a first-time mum who is concerned about the risks of the measles, mumps and rubella (MMR) vaccine. Her health visitor explains the health benefits of the vaccine.

1. What do you think the health visitor might say regarding the benefits of the MMR vaccine?
2. What might the health visitor say regarding the risks of contracting measles?

MMR (measles, mumps and rubella) immunisation programme, infection with measles is rare in the UK. However, some outbreaks have occurred because parents chose not to have their children immunised.

Hepatitis B

Hepatitis B virus (HBV) results in a serious disease that can cause liver failure and death. It is transmitted via blood and body fluids. As infection of the liver worsens, the individual will become jaundiced (skin becomes yellowy including the whites of the eyes) and nausea and vomiting are experienced.

Mumps

The virus (commonly a paramyxovirus) causes swelling and tenderness of the salivary glands. It usually affects children between 5 and 14 years of age, but can affect adults. Contaminated droplets enter the body via the mouth or nasal passages and the virus is also spread by saliva. The individual is infectious for approximately five days. Potential complications include infection of the inner ear (otitis media), nervous tissue and brain (encephalitis). Although rare, a complication of mumps is infertility.

Chickenpox and shingles

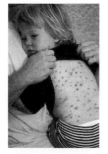

Chickenpox infection results in red, fluid-filled blisters all over the body

The virus *Herpes zoster* causes chickenpox in children and shingles in adults. It is mainly transmitted by droplets from an infected person. Chickenpox is typically a mild disease of childhood, however, in very young babies, teenagers, pregnant women and those with a weakened immune system, it can be more damaging. Complications include pneumonia (lung disease), conjunctivitis (eye inflammation) and encephalitis (inflammation of the brain). The symptoms include raised red spots surrounding a clear fluid centre, fever and tiredness. Later these form scabs and become itchy. Once you have had chickenpox, the virus lies dormant in the nerve roots of the spinal cord. It can be reactivated during adulthood if the immune system is weakened, resulting in shingles – a painful condition accompanied by a rash. If you have not had chickenpox as a child, you may catch it from someone with shingles.

Influenza (flu)

epidemic

widespread outbreak of disease that affects many people at one time

Influenza is caused by a virus that is continually changing or mutating, making it impossible for the body to develop immunity. It is spread by droplets, especially during coughing and sneezing. Every so often, the flu virus causes **epidemics**, usually in the winter. Symptoms include shivering, aching limbs, a high temperature, sore throat, cough and runny nose. There may also be vomiting and diarrhoea. These symptoms can last for up to three weeks and more, leaving the individual feeling very tired and sometimes depressed. Seasonal flu is estimated to kill several thousand people in the UK each year; the elderly are particularly vulnerable. Anti-flu vaccines are widely available each October or November. These will protect against certain types, and are thought to be highly if not fully effective.

Viral gastro-enteritis

Enteritis means inflammation of the large intestine, and *gastritis* means inflammation of the stomach. Some viruses cause this condition via droplets through coughs, sneezes, vomiting and diarrhoea. This type of virus can spread very quickly in a contained community, such as a children's home. Symptoms include severe stomach pains, vomiting and/or diarrhoea, which may be bloody. Symptoms may not arise until a day or two after contracting the virus.

Norovirus

Also known as 'winter vomiting viruses' (high incidences in the winter), 'small round-structured viruses' or 'Norwalk-like viruses'. Spread is by contact with infected people or contaminated surfaces, or by contaminated food or water. It can affect people of any age and it is thought that approximately 1 million people in the UK are affected in any one year. Symptoms are nausea, vomiting and diarrhoea, possibly also a high temperature and aching limbs. It is important to isolate clients and ensure sufficient fluids to avoid the complication of dehydration. For more about isolation care, see page 50.

Glandular fever

Caused by the Epstein-Barr virus, this is transmitted via saliva and the mucus in the nose and throat. This virus affects certain white blood cells called B-lymphocytes; their role is to produce antibodies to fight disease and as they begin to multiply they cause swelling of the glands. A throat swab confirms diagnosis and the disease takes about one month to run its course. Antibiotics are ineffective against a viral infection, however if a bacterial tonsillitis should occur, it can be treated with antibiotics.

Viral meningitis

This is less severe than the bacterial form and does not respond to antibiotics. It will run its course with similar symptoms, but the victim may experience headaches and tiredness for some weeks.

Activity 13

Complete a table like the one below for the viral infections you have studied in this section. Then research at least two other viral diseases and add this information to the table.

Disease	Transmission method	Symptoms	Complications

Fungi

Structure and properties

Fungi are non-motile multicellular organisms that were once thought to belong to the animal world (their genetic material is more closely related to animals, and they do have to feed off other material in order to live). Fungi include yeasts, moulds, mildews, toadstools and mushrooms. They reproduce via spores that grow into fungi as conditions become favourable. Some are useful to us, for example yeasts are used in making bread and beer, and certain moulds are used in the production and maturing of blue cheeses.

Moulds on foodstuffs will occur as food is ageing and this includes food at low temperatures, for example in fridges and cold-storage units. Moulds destroy food and are called spoilage organisms. Although they do not cause food poisoning they will make food foul-tasting. Mould affects food such as bread, oranges, lemons and cakes, and is often seen as white, green or black furry deposits. Occasionally fungal toxins can cause food-borne disease; a common problem with animal feed.

Yeasts prefer acidic environments and will happily grow in high sugar concentrations. They can be found in jam, honey, meats, wines and, occasionally, home-brewed beers. Yeasts do not normally cause food poisoning, but can cause mild stomach upsets.

The conditions fungi cause

Fungal infections in the UK are largely skin infections. All fungi like warm, moist conditions, so individuals should avoid wearing tight-fitting clothes, particularly if they tend to sweat a lot. Treatment is with anti-fungal creams and good personal hygiene.

Thrush

Thrush is caused by the fungus *Candida albicans* and is most often experienced as an infection of the vagina. However, in elderly people or young babies it can also be seen as little white spots on the tongue. This illustrates the vulnerability of these groups in society. Vaginal thrush can be spread by sexual intercourse. In males, the fungus on the penis is called *balanitis*, and is characterised by white itchy spots. Thrush can easily be treated. Thrush can arise due to prolonged use of antibiotics, which destroy bacteria but not fungal organisms. In the absence of bacteria, *Candida albicans* can thrive.

Ringworm (*Tinea*)

Despite its name this condition has nothing to do with worms. The fungus is often transmitted by contact with animals or other people with the condition. Areas affected are the scalp, the feet, nails, armpits, genital areas and the groin. There are different types of ringworm according to the area affected. *Tinea barbae* is ringworm of the face and neck and used to be known as 'barber's itch'. *Tinea corporis* affects the skin on the body and appears in some cases as advancing red rings. However an accurate diagnosis must be made to distinguish it from certain types of eczema, as treatment is different. The affected area grows outwards in a ring structure, causing redness and itching.

Athlete's foot (*Tinea pedis*)

Because fungi are saprophytes (they digest dead cells), they like sweaty feet and will eat up these cells, usually between the toes, though the heels can also be affected. This causes red, itchy and peeling skin. If left untreated, athlete's foot may destroy healthy tissue beneath these dead skin cells, leading to further irritation and soreness.

Jock itch (*Tinea cruris*)

This condition is characterised by red skin extending from the groin to the thighs which may cause chafing. Anti-fungal creams may help as well as keeping the legs clean, dry and avoiding skin surfaces touching.

Fungal nails (*Tinea unguium*)

Also known as *Onychomycosis*, this condition is characterised by thick yellow finger and toe nails, which also may be crumbly. There is treatment available for this condition.

If you observe a fungal condition in someone you are caring for, you should report what you see. Do not just apply any creams or ointments that you think might work, because the diagnosis of a fungal infection has to be accurate for the treatment to be effective. Avoiding warm and sweaty skin, however, and keeping areas clean and dry is good practice in any care environment and with all people you care for.

Care scenario: Leila

Leila has come to you because she has been diagnosed with a thrush infection. She is very embarrassed by the condition, and asks you what this means.

1. How will you explain to Leila what thrush is?
2. What advice will you give to Leila about how to prevent a thrush infection in the future?

Activity 14

You work in a nursing home. Your manager has asked you to be on the alert for fungal infections among the clients. What should you look out for?

Parasites

How different parasites affect the human body

A parasite is a plant or animal that lives on another organism in order to gain its nourishment and continued survival. The simplest kind of parasite is a very tiny single-celled life form called protozoa. These cause malaria (see page 5) and amoebic dysentery.

Parasites survive by attaching themselves in various ways to the human body, often originating by the hatching of larvae or eggs on the skin, hair or in the intestines.

Fleas (*Ctenocephalides*)

These are tiny insects without wings that lay eggs in narrow cracks and feed off human blood. They do not cause disease but do leave small itchy red spots. The eggs will not live for long if cleaning is regularly carried out.

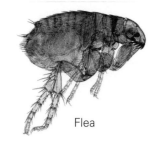

Flea

Lice (*Pediculosis capitis*)

Lice feed by sucking blood from their host's scalp many times a day, leaving little red marks that itch. Their eggs are small and white and stick very firmly to a hair shaft; they are easy to see and are commonly known as nits. The lice are spread easily by head-to-head contact with an infected person and controlled by regular conditioner or special lotion from the chemist. They cannot be removed simply by washing. The whole family must be treated for infection. Pubic lice are crab-shaped and spread during sexual contact.

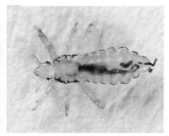

Head louse

Threadworms (*Strongyloides stercoralis*)

Threadworm is the most common worm infection, mostly found in children. The worms are tiny white threads about 1 cm long that live in the large intestine. The female lays her eggs on the skin around the anus, causing itching and irritation. During scratching, the tiny eggs are caught up in the fingernails and ingested when the hands are put in the mouth, before hatching in the large bowel (colon and rectum). The whole family must be treated for infection.

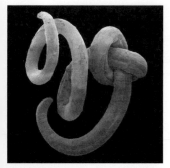

Threadworm

Scabies (*Sarcoptes sabiei*)

These creatures burrow in the outer skin layer, laying their eggs as they travel along. The indication of scabies is a red itchy rash that is quite scaly. It commonly affects the area between the fingers, the wrists, buttocks, lower arms and armpits. The mites are transmitted by crawling from one infected person to another. The whole family must be treated for infection.

Scabies

Bed bugs (*Cimex lectularius*)

These tiny insects live in bedding and tiny cracks in bedrooms. They are generally only active at night, when they feed off the blood of their host, however they are no longer common.

Tapeworm (*Taenia solium*)

Tapeworm is a ribbon-shaped parasite that lives in the intestines of people or animals. The worm is ingested as a result of eating a tapeworm cyst (found on undercooked pork or beef) or after contact with infected animals. The head of the tapeworm attaches itself to the lining of the intestine by means of suckers. Segments of the worm are produced continually, since the worm is effectively absorbing digested food and growing bigger; they can grow up to 9 metres (30 feet) in length. The head of the worm has to be removed in order for the whole thing to be expelled; this is done by taking certain drugs.

Tapeworm are not common in the UK but exist quite frequently in warmer developing countries. Care must be taken when visiting these countries to ensure that only thoroughly cooked meat is eaten.

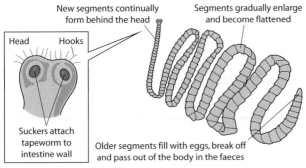

New segments continually form behind the head

Segments gradually enlarge and become flattened

Head   Hooks

Suckers attach tapeworm to intestine wall

Older segments fill with eggs, break off and pass out of the body in the faeces

Tapeworm

1. Referring to the properties and structure of a bacterium, what helps it to grow and multiply?

2. How does a virus start its pathway to illness?

3. Describe how mould affects food.

4. Name four types of parasite. Describe how each of these parasites invades and lives off humans.

5. What are the differences between viruses and bacteria?

6. What is a saprophyte?

7. What happens to bacteria when conditions become unfavourable?

8. What are spores? How can they be destroyed?

The chain of infection can be broken at any stage to prevent infection. To understand how best to do this, you need to know what pathogens require in order to grow, multiply and spread. You also need to be aware of the common routes of transmission, for example direct contact, droplets, flies, hands, fomites, faeces, air, dust, food and water.

Activity 15

Think back to what you learned earlier about the chain of infection. Identify the different stages by which transient pathogens succeed in causing infection.

_____

_____

_____

_____

What you need to learn

- How pathogenic micro-organisms grow
- How pathogenic micro-organisms spread

How pathogenic micro-organisms grow

Conditions required for growth

As you saw on page 19, in order to grow and multiply, bacteria need:

- nutrients (food, minerals)
- oxygen (although anaerobic bacteria survive without oxygen)
- warmth
- moisture
- most, but not all, prefer a neutral environment (neither acid nor alkaline)
- time for these conditions to remain stable.

Some bacteria produce spores that can lie dormant for years and become activated (produce pathogenic microbes) when conditions become favourable.

A **reservoir** is an area that contains pathogenic micro-organisms. It could be a pond, a dishcloth, items of food, a wound or waste matter such as urine or faeces – any place where conditions are favourable for growth. The reservoir that causes most concern is unclean hands.

reservoir

area that contains pathogenic micro-organisms and provides the right conditions for their growth

Where do we find micro-organisms?

The bacterium *Staphylococcus aureas* lives on the hands of around 40 per cent of the population. Other transient pathogens attach themselves to skin cells and can survive for several hours, days or weeks. They may be transferred to surfaces or washed away by good cleaning or disinfection.

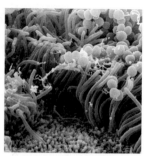

Staphylococcus bacteria in the nose; these may be spread via the hands, or by sneezes

Care scenario: Mary

Mary has been asked to empty the urine catheter bag of an individual in her care. She chats to the individual while she carries out the task. When Mary has finished, she tidies up and makes sure the individual is comfortable. Then she goes to serve breakfast to a different client in another room. Because Mary is running a little late, she does not bother to wash her hands before moving on to the next client.

1. Describe the risks Mary's actions pose for herself, the second client and other individuals in the care setting.

   _____

   _____

2. How would you explain to Mary that her actions are dangerous and inform her of the need to prevent cross-infection?

   _____

   _____

Activity 16

Complete the table below by stating how each term is important for the growth and spread of pathogens.

Term	Role in growth and spread of pathogens
Reservoir	
Nutrients	
Time	
Warmth	
Moisture	
Oxygen	

What do you do in your care routines to help people develop a stronger immune system?

How pathogenic micro-organisms spread

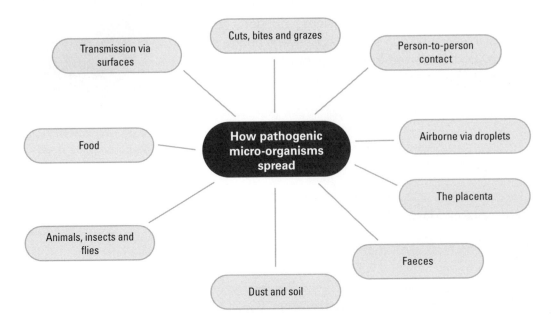

Person-to-person contact

Infections that are spread from person to person include ringworm and the *Herpes zoster* and chickenpox viruses. Skin infections are commonly transmitted through direct contact.

Unprotected sexual contact with an infected person can result in the transfer of micro-organisms via body fluids, for example semen or vaginal secretions. Herpes, gonorrhoea and chlamydia are sexual diseases that are currently on the increase.

Cuts, grazes and bites

Micro-organisms can enter the bloodstream directly via contaminated needles, cuts and grazes on the skin or damaged mucous membranes inside the body. Insects and animals may infect the blood by bites and the injecting of toxins. Remember, because the blood circulates, a localised infection can soon become a systemic infection.

Transmission via surfaces

Some bacteria will remain on the fur of animals, in dust particles or on food (especially in a warm room). From there, they can be transferred to other surfaces or inside the body by direct contact (for example hand to mouth). It is also possible to become infected via indirect contact with fomites (see page 18), for example the infected person's handkerchief, mobile telephone or towel.

Airborne via droplets

Droplets are tiny fragments of infected mucus. A sneeze can hurl 20,000 droplets of moisture containing bacteria and viruses a distance of more than 4 metres (13 feet). This also happens during coughing. Once airborne, the micro-organisms can be inhaled by another person, causing respiratory infection. The droplets often settle onto surfaces and then dry out, leaving the pathogens to contaminate the next person who touches the surface. Colds are often spread by hands contaminated in this way.

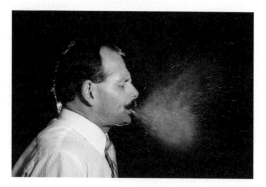

The spray from a sneeze can be highly contagious

Activity 17

1 What types of pathogens could be expelled in a sneeze?

_____

_____

_____

2 If the influenza virus were expelled in a sneeze, what conditions would contribute to a widespread epidemic?

_____

_____

_____

Care scenario: Lucy

Mrs Andrews has been admitted to the nursing home with a large bed sore on her buttock. Her main carer, Lucy, has come to work today with a heavy cold. As she changes Mrs Andrews's sheets, she sneezes, uses her handkerchief and places this loosely up her long sleeve. Then she proceeds to roll Mrs Andrews on to a clean sheet.

1. Describe the possible faults in this process.
2. Explain how Mrs Andrews may become contaminated by pathogenic organisms.
3. What procedure should Lucy have followed?
4. What infection is common in hospitals and homes? Why do you think this is?

Food

Food can contain pathogens at any stage of the production process, from raw meat through to storage and after cooking.

- Raw meat can be contaminated, for example chicken might be home to campylobacter and salmonella, which cause food poisoning. If the cooking time is not long enough or the temperature not hot enough, the food will still contain the organisms when it is served. The ideal core temperature to reach and attain for a minimum of 3 minutes is 75 degrees Celsius.

- If meat or cook–chill products are stored in a refrigerator that is set at too high a temperature, organisms may start to multiply. (Fridges should be set between 0 and 5 degrees Celsius.)

Activity 18

1 Why is food labelled with 'best-before' and 'use-by' dates?

_____

_____

2 List the measures to prevent food poisoning and gastro-enteric infections. Make your list as comprehensive as possible.

_____

_____

Animals, insects and flies

All animals, insects and flies carry organisms, some more harmful than others. You may recall the example of how the Anopheles mosquito causes malaria (see page 5). Flies are frequently found in dirty areas, for example eating old decayed food or animal faeces. Later on, if they land on your meal and vomit, they will leave behind thousands of pathogens. Bacteria can also be deposited via tiny hairs on their legs.

Certain insects or snakes may bite, injecting toxins into the bloodstream. This is commonly referred to as blood poisoning or septicaemia. Snake bites are rarely a problem in the UK.

Dust and soil

Dust can contain spores. Although spores can remain dormant (inactive) for a long time, favourable conditions just like the ones you have read about may trigger germination (growth and multiplication).

Often organisms found in soil are anaerobic (they dislike oxygen). Root vegetables, such as carrots and beetroot, and salad vegetables that are unwashed may harbour pathogens.

Faeces

Faeces are highly contaminated. Pathogens are excreted in human faeces and can easily be transferred to hands during toilet visits or when attending to clients' needs. Dog and cat faeces may carry roundworm; ingested roundworm eggs can cause fever and eye damage in children. This is just one reason why there are fines in the UK for people who allow their dogs to foul public areas.

The placenta

The placenta feeds the unborn baby in the womb, but pathogenic micro-organisms may also pass to the developing child. Pregnant women therefore have to take special care of the following:

- Some lambs are born carrying the germs that cause listeriosis, toxoplasmosis and chlamydia. These could be transmitted to the unborn child, so it is essential for pregnant women to stay away at lambing time.

- Toxoplasmosis can be contracted by contact with cat faeces, so another precaution is for pregnant women to avoid litter trays and to wear gloves when gardening.

- Listeriosis can be contracted via certain foods, so pregnant women are advised to avoid soft cheeses, pâtés and cold meats, and to wash all fruit and vegetables.

- Rubella, if contracted in the first 12 weeks of pregnancy, can cause irreparable damage to the growing foetus, resulting in disabilities after birth.

- HIV can be transmitted to the developing foetus in pregnancy.

Care scenario: Listeriosis

In 1989 the UK government issued a warning to risk groups such as pregnant women and the immune-suppressed to avoid soft cheeses, cook–chill produce and pâté. These products were found to carry the organism *Listeria monocytogenes* which causes the food-borne disease listeriosis. This bacteria can multiply in low temperatures. Listeriosis can cause miscarriage and even meningitis.

1. Why are the foods listed more likely to carry the bacteria *Listeria monocytogenes*?
2. What steps could be taken in your setting to prevent individuals coming into contact with this bacterium?

Activity 19

How do you ensure in your daily duties that infection from the following contaminants does not occur?

1. Dust:
   _____
   _____

2. Flies:
   _____
   _____

3. Blood:
   _____
   _____

4. Faeces:
   _____
   _____

5. Urine:
   _____
   _____

6. Nasal mucus/sputum:
   _____
   _____

Activity 20

Tick the following statements to indicate whether you think each is true or false.

	True	False
1. A respiratory infection is more likely to be caught from unprotected sex		
2. After a chicken pie has stood at room temperature for 4 hours it will not contain micro-organisms		
3. If you wear disposable gloves when in contact with blood and body fluids there is no need to wash your hands		
4. Pathogenic bacteria can grow in cold temperatures		
5. A virus divides by a process known as binary fission		
6. Flagella is the name for the head of a bacterium		
7. A fomite is an inanimate object contaminated with pathogenic bacteria		
8. HIV can only be transmitted via blood		

1. Describe how a bacterium multiplies.

2. What conditions are needed for bacteria to spread?

3. Describe the properties of a spore.

4. Describe how a virus multiplies.

5. Explain the difference between direct and indirect contamination.

6. Explain at least five routes of transmission of pathogenic organisms.

2

Preventing and controlling the spread of infection

2.1 Understand the standard precautions to prevent infection and its spread

Standard **precautions** to prevent infection and its spread are detailed in organisational policies and procedures. These help staff in care homes, hospitals and residential settings to keep the risks of infection as low as possible. It is absolutely vital to keep preventive measures such as good hygiene practices consistent and of the highest standard at all times. Just now and then is unacceptable and will allow pathogens momentum for growth.

precautions
safety measures to protect against possible danger, illness or injury

You should be able to relate much of your practice to the principles and procedures that are described and explained in this section.

What you need to learn

- The principles of hand hygiene
- The importance of appropriate personal protective equipment (PPE)
- General cleanliness
- Principles of isolation nursing
- The part immunisation plays in infection control
- Safe practice procedures
- Management of outbreaks of infection

You need to continually be aware of the necessity of regular and thorough hand-washing. Any duties about to be performed involving contact with individuals, food, materials and equipment possibly contaminated with pathogens should trigger the need to do a thorough hand-wash. Try to make this an unconscious regular habit, i.e. something you do automatically.

The principles of hand hygiene

The role of the hands as a route of transmission in the UK is poorly understood by the general public. As a result many people fail to wash their hands to an acceptable standard. Small cracks on the hands can harbour pathogenic microbes such as MRSA.

Recent research in the United States found that when a programme of vigorous hand-washing was introduced in care homes there was a 33 per cent reduction in common colds and a 50 per cent reduction in diarrhoea.

A good hand-washing technique

- Use warm running water to wet the hands.
- Use around 3–5 ml (a teaspoon) of good quality unperfumed liquid soap to work up lather.

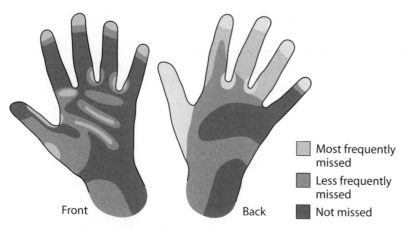

	Most frequently missed
	Less frequently missed
	Not missed

Front   Back

Areas commonly missed during hand-washing. Note that the most frequently missed areas are the thumbs and fingertips and inter-digital spaces

- Ensure the fingers (including tips), thumbs and wrists, including the insides, are massaged well with soap lather and digits interlocking. The process should take *at least* 20 seconds (longer for heavily soiled hands).
- Rinse thoroughly in warm running water.
- Dry with a paper towel.
- Use a foot-operated bin to dispose of the paper towel.

Activity 21

List the times and circumstances when you should do a thorough hand-wash while carrying out your duties.

Alcohol gels can disinfect hands that are not heavily contaminated, but they do not clean. Lotions should contain anti-microbial properties, as some lotions may support the growth of pathogens. Non-water-based hand hygiene agents based on isopropyl alcohol formulated into a gel or lotion are now widely used for speedy disinfection of the hands after visits to the toilet, before serving food, in between client care and after bed changing.

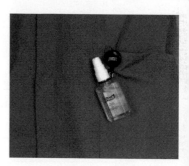

Alcohol gels disinfect hands after washing, but are not a substitute for thorough washing

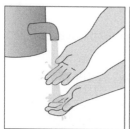

1. Wet hands with running water.

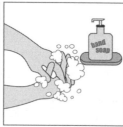

2. Rub hands together with soap and lather well, covering all surfaces.

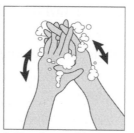

3. Weave fingers and thumbs together and slide them back and forth.

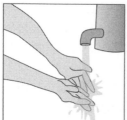

4. Rinse hands under a stream of clean, running water until all soap is gone.

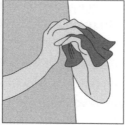

5. Blot hands dry with clean towel.

How to wash your hands thoroughly

Equipment and facilities to support hand hygiene

Disposable gloves

Latex and non-latex (some people are allergic to latex) disposable gloves are worn for procedures that could be high risk, i.e. involving wounds, body fluids and discharges.

An example of a procedure requiring disposable gloves would be the insertion of pessaries or suppositories. Catheterisation, however, requires sterile gloves. Gloves are an important barrier and protect the client from our potential pathogens as well as protecting carers from the client's potential pathogens. The combination of donning aprons and gloves and good hand hygiene constitutes the practice of 'universal precautions'. Procedures are performed aseptically, which means no contact with any possible contaminant.

Activity 22: Universal precautions

Catheterisation is an invasive procedure requiring the use of sterile gloves. List three other procedures that you think also need the use of 'universal precautions' and explain why.

Procedure using universal precautions	Reason for an aseptic technique

Wearing gloves is no substitute for washing hands. This must still be done as stated in the guidelines on pages 44–45, and should be repeated after carefully removing and disposing of the gloves. This means not touching contaminated gloves with your hands.

Facilities for hand hygiene

- There should be a sufficient number of wash basins available, positioned at regular intervals.
- Taps should be non-hand-operated and running water of suitable temperature.
- Liquid soap and/or alcohol gels should be kept in plentiful supply.
- Paper towels or hand driers should be easily accessible close to the wash basin. Hand driers should be quick and effective. Walking away with residue moisture on hands could be an opportunity for cross-contamination because damp surfaces transfer micro-organisms better than dry ones.
- Keeping wash basins clean is essential. There is nothing worse than having to wash your hands in a dirty basin with a bar of soap that is old and cracked – the chances are this will not be an effective process.

Activity 23

You have been asked to monitor the cleanliness and availability of the hand-washing facilities in your setting. Create a checklist of what to look for so other staff can also check.

The importance of appropriate personal protective equipment (PPE)

Personal protective equipment (PPE) refers to uniforms including any protective head covering, gloves and aprons. You should change into these when you arrive for duty or if uniform becomes contaminated during a shift. You should also remove any jewellery and ensure there are no loose parts on your uniform.

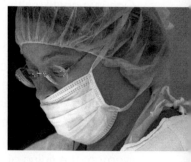

Nurse wearing a mask in the correct position

If you are laundering your own uniform you should be given instructions on the appropriate temperature in which to wash your garment. Usually this is 60 degrees Celsius.

If you are dealing with contaminated dressings, body fluids and blood, or if you go into a room where an individual is being barrier nursed, disposable aprons and gloves should be worn. Immediately after disposal of materials, aprons and gloves should be placed into yellow 'high risk' bags and hands washed thoroughly. Soiled uniforms should be changed immediately and aprons worn only once per individual.

Other PPE may include masks, visors or goggles. After each use these should be cleaned or disposed of in accordance with manufacturers' instructions.

Activity 24

1. Why should you change into your uniform when you arrive for duty?

2. Why should you remove jewellery and check for loose parts on your uniform?

3. How does wearing a mask or goggles minimise the risk of infection?

General cleanliness

Personal

It follows from what you have explored so far that in order to avoid infection, you need to maintain high standards of personal hygiene. This primarily means daily washing and good drying followed by dressing in clean clothes. Uniforms should only be used for one shift and changed if stained with a possible contaminant. If you become ill you must report this to your manager, and if you have gastro-intestinal symptoms you must not go to work. The Occupational Health Department must be informed and advice taken.

Your client's personal cleanliness and care of effects

A large part of your role is to ensure the personal cleanliness of the people you care for. When bathing the client or assisting them to wash and bathe, ensure that the face is cleaned with a separate cloth and towels are separate for the upper and lower parts of the body. Take care when cleaning around catheters, using swabs once only. Check that catheters are not blocked or a source of irritation, particularly with post-menopausal women: the lining of the urethra is thinned and more likely to become infected and damaged. If you are washing groin and vaginal areas, wipe once from front to back to avoid bacteria being pushed into the urethra.

Ensure a good supply of tissues, urinals and containers with lids for sputum collection. Dispose of these regularly and thoroughly wash hands, finishing with an alcohol rub.

Check that clients have clean clothes to wear and that finger and toe nails are clean and regularly clipped. Discuss any issues of concern with your manager, for example if you think something you have noticed needs a medical opinion or perhaps the services of a chiropodist.

Environment, equipment and materials

Every area within a care setting requires identification of hazards and risks. This involves:

- risk assessment
- planning
- monitoring
- documenting
- ordering
- evaluating (is everything working efficiently?).

Risk assessment

A risk assessment will consider such things as the design of the setting, the building materials used, how often to clean areas, and which kind of spillages and contamination may occur. It also looks at the safe disposal of spillages and waste products (see also page 71). Daily routines would also be considered, to determine whether they contribute to effective infection control. Areas are assessed as low risk, medium risk and high risk. Issues that may be identified include:

- Risks created by materials such as flooring, walls and work surfaces. Cracks and damp may indicate an infection risk since pathogens could gather here.
- Cracked tiles and peeling paint will require replacing as these would be hazardous if scrubbing were to take place.

When in contact with vulnerable people:

- your skin should be free of lesions (wounds) and any cut covered with a blue waterproof plaster, especially when duties involve serving food.
- your nails should be short and should not be bitten
- your shoes should be sensible and not open-toed
- your oral (mouth) hygiene should be good, e.g. regular tooth-brushing
- if not worn short, your hair should be tied back away from the face
- you must seek medical advice if you have any skin irritations
- you should report stomach upsets to Occupational Health, follow advice and do not work.

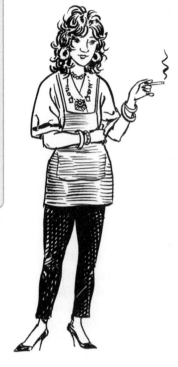

Activity 25

This care worker will be assisting you in your duties. Explain to her the need to dress more appropriately using the information in this section.

- Clinical areas and theatres will require a deeper and more frequent cleaning schedule. Equipment here should be sterilised by autoclaving or other methods (see also page 62).
- Sluices will be considered high risk and demand special attention.
- In areas where food is served a specific system is used to identify potential hazards. This is called HACCP (hazard analysis and critical control point).

Risk assessment is further described in Unit 4.3.

Planning

This is about delivering the correct courses of action based on the risk assessment. Plans need to be agreed and consistently followed by all staff on rotating shifts.

Monitoring the environment and equipment

It is important to attend to soiled or worn equipment and materials. Storage of equipment should ensure that sterilised packages are away from non-sterile items and that packaging has not been damaged. Discard any damaged packs.

Documenting

Documenting is about recording all of the steps you have taken to deal with hazards and risks in the care environment. All items cleaned or disposed of must be listed, with details of when this was done and signatures to confirm such actions.

Ordering

New containers of cleaning materials must be ordered before they run out. In the community, ordering may involve more sterile supplies, waste bags or boxes, sharps bins for self-medicating patients or urinary/continence products.

Activity 26

Describe how your duties ensure that you work from clean areas and tasks to dirty ones.

Principles of isolation nursing

isolation

a method of physical protection by caring for an individual (who has a specific infection requiring this type of care) away from other vulnerable people and using equipment, materials and processes of care specifically for them

If an individual in your care is thought to be infectious they must be placed in a single room. This is known as being placed in **isolation**. Isolation is also required for very sick people who are immuno-suppressed. If a single room is not available an infected person must be cared for with other infected people and the room or area kept as isolated and separate as possible with the principles of universal precautions strictly adhered to.

There are two types of isolation nursing:

Source isolation segregates the infected person to prevent the spread of infection to other patients.

Protective isolation segregates the susceptible person to prevent them from acquiring an infection from other people.

With the exception of used bedpans or urinals, any materials or objects that are taken into the room must stay there until the infection has passed. Wherever possible, disposable articles should be used. It is useful to keep a plentiful supply of bedpans/urinals in the room. You must wear disposable gowns or aprons, and gloves that are only applied after washing the hands thoroughly. Separate gloves must be worn when dealing with blood, urine or faeces. If the infection is airborne, masks must also be worn and bed linen not shaken during changing. Any regular items to help with the care and treatment of the individual should remain in the room and be disinfected or discarded after use. It is useful to have signage on the door telling visitors to check with the duty officer or nurse in charge before entering.

Waste

Infectious waste is placed in yellow bags that are labelled as such and contaminated bed linen is placed in separate laundry bags marked 'infective', usually red. (See page 71 for the newly revised procedures for disposal of clinical waste.) A wash basin should be in the room and paper towels should be provided for hand-drying. A foot-operated bin should be next to the wash basin for waste.

Care scenario: Preparation for isolation

You have been asked to check out and prepare a single room for Mr Black, who has MRSA and an open wound.

What provision will you make for Mr Black and care staff so you can ensure safe, hygienic procedures and control of infection?

The importance of care sector workers being free from infection

Care workers must be protected against possible blood-borne infections. A common immunisation programme involves protection against hepatitis B (see page 30). However, not all organisations will offer this protection as the threat may be deemed low risk.

It is necessary to carry out a risk assessment before gowning up and wearing masks for infections that may not need this procedure. For example, giving a cup of tea will pose no risks to the infected person or the carer. The infected or vulnerable person's dignity must be considered. Part of your role as a carer is to dispel any myths and reassure clients and visitors that high standards of control are to everyone's benefit.

Your local Occupational Health Department will advise on any personal illness that may pose a threat to individuals and staff. It also organises the screening (checking) of potential carriers of **notifiable diseases** and may organise examination of infected faeces, which must go to a laboratory. If food-borne infection is suspected, the regional Director of Public Health should be contacted and samples of food, vomit and/or faeces retained for examination.

notifiable disease

*disease that needs reporting to the appropriate authorities. Examples of notifiable diseases are those that may cause epidemic or **pandemic** outbreaks, including smallpox and anthrax*

pandemic

epidemic over a wide area, i.e. a major outbreak of disease affecting people in many different countries at the same time

How do occupational health departments link with public health? Research reported incidents of infection in your region and discover how they were managed.

Activity 27

1. Who may pose a threat to individuals who need isolation nursing because they are vulnerable to infections?

2. What will you do to minimise these risks?

The part immunisation plays in infection control

What is immunisation?

Immunisation works by creating protection against pathogens. There are two types of immunisation:

The first type involves introducing a tiny amount of a pathogen into the bloodstream (usually by injection). This prompts the body to produce antibodies, so that exposure to large numbers of the antigen in the future will trigger the appropriate antibody to fight the pathogens, thereby preventing disease. This type is called *active immunisation.*

The second type is referred to as *passive* – artificially made antibodies designed to give short-term protection, as in the case of the influenza vaccine. Vulnerable people receive this annually.

Childhood immunisations

In the UK there is a programme of immunisation from early infancy. The table below lists the routine immunisations offered to children in the UK.

> Choose two of the immunisations listed below and carry out research into the diseases they provide protection against.

Routine immunisation schedule for children in the UK (Source: NHS Immunisation Information website, 2006)

Age of child	Immunisations offered
Birth (only in babies at risk)	• Tuberculosis
2 months	• '5-in-1': Diphtheria; Pertussis (Whooping Cough); Tetanus; Polio; Haemophilus influenzae type B (Hib) • Pneumococcal conjugate vaccine (PCV)
3 months	• '5-in-1' (as above) • Meningitis C (meningococcal group C)
4 months	• '5-in-1' (as above) • Meningitis C (meningococcal group C) • Pneumococcal conjugate vaccine (PCV)
12 months (approx)	• Meningitis C (meningococcal group C) • Haemophilus Influenzae type B (Hib)
Around 13 months (approx)	• Measles, Mumps and Rubella (MMR) • Pneumococcal conjugate vaccine (PCV)
Pre-school (between 3 years 4 months and 5 years)	• Diphtheria; Pertussis (Whooping Cough); Tetanus; Polio • Measles, Mumps and Rubella (MMR)
13 to 18 years old	• Diphtheria; Tetanus; Polio (given by school nurse or the local health centre)

Care scenario: Rubella

Rubella is a mild viral infection that can affect anyone of any age. However, if a pregnant woman were to catch it, the virus would damage her unborn child. In 1969, a vaccination against rubella was developed. Today, the majority of people in the UK are vaccinated against rubella between 12 to 15 months of age and then again at around 4 years. The vaccine hopefully provides lifelong protection.

1. Why do you think a second 'booster' vaccination is needed at 4 years?

   _____

   _____

2. What are the advantages of immunising 'the majority of the people in the UK' against rubella?

   _____

   _____

Immunisation for travel

Diseases that have been almost wiped out in the West are often widespread in developing countries, for example in parts of Africa, Asia and South America. Before travelling abroad it is advisable to check with your local health centre or a specialist travel clinic about immunisations required to visit certain countries. For example, if travelling to a developing country you may be advised to be vaccinated against cholera, yellow fever and hepatitis B. To guard against malaria, a course of tablets may be given a few weeks before and after travel, so the body has time to develop immunity.

What immunisations have you had, either as a child or for travel? Did you experience any side-effects?

Activity 28

Complete the table below by carrying out research into the immunisations required before travelling to the following countries.

Country	Travel immunisations required
Dominican Republic	
India	
Kenya	

Safe practice procedures

How to prevent sharps injuries and dispose of sharps safely

'Sharps' are anything with the potential to cut the skin. They can include needles, scalpels, stitch cutters and glass ampoules. Safe procedures involve the prevention of cross-contamination via blood, for example HIV and hepatitis B infection.

According to an audit by the Department of Health (2003), there were 1550 incidents of blood-borne virus contact in the healthcare sector between July 1997 and June 2002. Following training, healthcare assistants are able to give subcutaneous injections (just under the skin) and may assist nurses with intra-muscular and intra-venous injections. It is essential not to pass these needles from hand to hand and to check they are not broken.

After a sharp is used you must:

- not re-sheath it but place it in a designated container (see the notes on Safe disposal of healthcare waste regulations, November 2006)
- check that containers are not more than two-thirds full
- check that containers are not accessible to the general public
- check that there are sufficient disposable trays for moving used sharps.

Clients self-medicating in their own homes should be provided with their own sharps bins (yellow rigid containers with yellow or purple lids) and informed about the risks regarding contamination.

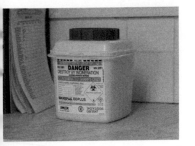

Used sharps must be placed in a sharps bin

How to handle and serve food safely

Healthcare staff involved in the serving of food must check that their uniform and/or PPE (see page 47) has not been contaminated by earlier procedures. If there is any doubt, they must wear a clean apron. It is very important that hands are washed thoroughly (see pages 44–45) before handling food. You must also ensure no coughing or sneezing.

Another important consideration is to check that hot food is indeed piping hot and cold food is chilled. (Warm temperatures are ideal for the growth of pathogens.) To protect from airborne microbes and flies, food should always be covered, either with an insulating lid or clingfilm for cold food.

Individuals receiving food should be given the opportunity to wash their hands. This may involve assistance from a member of staff. This is not only a prevention procedure – it also makes the client feel clean and comfortable prior to meals.

Disposal of uneaten food should be immediate. It should be placed in a covered bin in a safe area that has been chosen specially for the purpose. The selected area must be free from pests and accessible to refuse collectors.

Care scenario: Changing linen

You are about to be involved in giving out lunches in a care home. You have just finished changing bed linen.

Describe the sequence you follow and the checks you make, from the bed change to collecting lunches on trays and serving them to clients in bed.

How to manage soiled dressings

It is absolutely essential to wear disposable gloves and aprons when attending to wounds or soiled beds. Keeping clean equipment, instruments and linen away from soiled articles is vital in the prevention of infection. Organisations vary in their procedures for this management. Currently nearly all organisations have yellow bags for clinical waste, however the colour-coded system of clinical waste disposal was revised in January 2007; waste for incineration which includes soiled dressings will be orange, with offensive, non-infectious healthcare waste being disposed of in yellow bags or black bags with yellow stripes. As these guidelines are very new, staff should seek guidance for their particular organisation from the waste-management contractor or the infection control team (see the table on page 71).

Whether you work in a residential home, in a care home or in someone's own home, suspected infectious dressings are disposed of in orange clinical waste bags and are collected for incineration. It is the healthcare worker's responsibility to ensure the collector is aware of the contents and how to transport and dispose of them to reduce potential hazards.

> Remember, objects can become contaminated by direct contact.

Management of soiled laundry

It is essential to keep soiled linen separate from other linen. Soiled linen is placed in red alginate bags that disintegrate (break down) in a high-temperature wash. You will need to wear disposable gloves when handling soiled linen and dispose of the gloves carefully.

Afterwards, wash your hands thoroughly and use an alcohol rub. Temperatures for washing soiled linen and bedclothes need to be higher than normal, in the range of 60–90 degrees Celsius.

In a care home people with identified infections have their own laundry cycle that is kept separate from other residents'. It is important that clothing is named. This is not important in a person's own home, but you should ensure strict separation of soiled laundry, sluicing off any faecal matter and washing at high temperatures to kill off pathogens.

In residential homes or in domiciliary care, people who are incontinent can receive help with specially designed products to protect the skin and to help minimise infections. An example of these is kyle pads, which are soft broad bed sheets that protect the area of the bed the client lies on. They are capable of being washed at high temperatures. Throughout the healthcare industry, specialised incontinence nurses will give advice on the best products and care available for clients who are incontinent.

One further point to bear in mind is that if off-site laundries are used, the collector needs to be aware of the infectious contents. Currently these are classified and packaged as UN 3291. Special bags are available for contaminated mattresses.

Care scenario: Safe procedures checklist

Your line manager asks you to help a new care assistant understand procedures for infection control.

Draw up and complete a chart like the one below, to help the care assistant understand why the following procedures are necessary.

Procedure	What to do	Why it is necessary
Sharps disposal		
Handling and serving of food		
Management of soiled dressings		
Management of soiled laundry		

Management of outbreaks of infection

There are a number of practices that organisations and individuals can adopt to prevent outbreaks of infection. These involve:

- continual attention to personal and environmental cleanliness
- strict procedures for the prevention of cross-contamination
- isolation of individuals with suspected or identified infectious disease

- thorough training for all staff on infection control
- regular meetings with infection control teams (groups of specialists who review practice and procedures in healthcare settings, monitor incidences of disease and conditions and are continually accessible for advice, whether preventive or during outbreaks)
- an efficient reporting and complaints procedure for staff, clients and visitors.

Organisations must follow laws and regulations. The Commission for Social Care Inspection (CSCI) has a duty to inspect all care homes to ensure high standards are maintained. (Laws and regulations are addressed on pages 64–73, and how organisations transfer these into policies and procedures is addressed in Unit 3.2.)

Environmental and public health departments inspect premises that have received complaints of poor practice or possible food poisoning. Investigations are carried out to include all possible contaminants including workers. Once doctors have identified an outbreak they will inform public health, whose role is to prevent and control infections as soon as they are notified.

1. Describe in detail how to thoroughly wash hands and use alcohol preparations.

2. What pathogen can be found on cuts, boils and skin lesions?

3. List the main points about effective personal and protective clothing.

4. Explain why cleaning schedules should be monitored.

5. Describe how artificial immunisation works.

6. What are the duties of the Occupational Health Department?

7. Describe how you would avoid a sharps injury.

8. Describe four principles of isolation nursing.

9. Describe four principles of food safety.

10. State six measures to prevent outbreaks of infection.

Carry out research into an outbreak of MRSA, *E. Coli* (as a food-borne organism) *Salmonella* or *Clostridium difficile*. How was the outbreak managed? What people and departments were involved?

1. What are the consequences for healthcare organisations when infection outbreaks are reported in the media?

2. How might the staff who work in these organisations feel?

It is illegal to fail to report incidences of possible food poisoning or food-borne illness.

If you are not careful when carrying out procedures for waste disposal you could undermine the hygiene control procedures you perform and those performed by others. This section looks at how to dispose of both household and clinical, or hazardous, waste safely. It also describes how to deal with biological spillages.

What you need to learn

- The safe disposal of household waste
- The safe disposal of clinical/hazardous waste
- How to deal with biological spillages

The safe disposal of household waste

All food waste must be placed in bin bags then put in a sturdy refuse bag before being placed in an outdoor bin. Indoor waste areas should be positioned away from clean areas and arranged in the most convenient place for easy disposal, for example without walking through food-preparation areas. Bins should be foot-operated and have secure fitting lids. As full bags are removed, bins should be wiped down with detergent.

These days we are strongly encouraged to recycle whatever we can and most local authorities provide suitable containers for plastic, garden rubbish, paper, cardboard and glass. Food and drink waste must be removed first before placing in the proper containers. Once emptied, containers should be cleaned out with very hot water and detergent.

Household waste is disposed of in black bags.

The safe disposal of clinical waste

The term clinical waste refers to blood, urine, vomit, sputum, faeces, wound dressings, contaminated pads, disposable aprons and gloves and small plastic disposable instruments. These are high-risk items and as such must be disposed of very carefully to avoid cross-infection. Local authorities collect this kind of waste for incineration (burning) and now provide orange plastic bags or boxes for the purpose. When full, the bags are stored in a safe area chosen especially for the purpose, ready for collection. It is important that risk assessments of waste disposal are carried out in order to comply with the safe disposal regulations of November 2006. Any advice can be provided by the infection control team or the waste management contractor.

Activity 29

You enter the sluice area to find a torn yellow bag with its contents spilled over the floor. Describe your actions.

_____

_____

Biological spillages

Any liquid that has the potential to contaminate objects or cause damage to skin or breathing is termed 'biological'. This includes blood, vomit and body fluids. Incorrect use of cleaning fluids, for example mixing them or not diluting to the correct strength, may result in the individual being affected by toxic fumes.

Cleaning fluids always carry a blue cross on a red background to inform you of the high risk of contamination. However there is now a range of warning symbols for categories of hazards. There should be clear written procedures that specify the reporting and investigation process that ensures a safe system of working. There should also be guidelines as to how waste can be safely cleared to decontaminate an area. The wearing of disposable gloves and aprons is paramount in minimising the risk of contamination.

If you are cleaning with hazardous substances you must comply with the Control of Substances Hazardous to Health (COSHH) Regulations 2002. These state that a risk assessment must be carried out before using hazardous substances, and that all staff must be fully trained in their use and control (see also pages 66–67).

Should a spillage occur it is essential to immediately dilute and mop the area until dry. You must wear gloves. However, if there is a risk of toxic inhalation you must leave the area immediately and inform management, who should then contact the regional environmental health department to seek advice. The introduction of risk assessment and COSHH (see pages 66–67) makes this scenario unlikely. If anybody experiences breathing difficulties then the emergency services should be called, by ringing either 999 or 112, and first aid given.

Disposal of waste is now categorised using colour coding (see page 71).

Hospitals and care homes have to be kept clean and high standards maintained throughout all areas and service provision. Some areas will need frequent dusting or cleaning but others carry a higher risk because of activities that are performed in that area, for example an operating theatre or in the case of dealing with contaminated waste, the sluice area. In both areas there is a constant need to significantly reduce the chances of contamination. Waste should never be allowed to build up in sluices, and bedpans and urinals should be macerated as soon as they are brought into the sluice. After disposal hands should be washed and alcohol rub applied. It is essential that all members of a team appreciate and practise frequent good cleaning techniques using hot water and detergent and disinfecting at regular times according to the risk assessment's recommendations.

If you work in someone's own home you should explain how and why you are carrying out a good cleaning schedule and advise the client to help maintain high standards. Mobile clients should be supplied with alcohol gels and caring for immobile clients will involve ensuring that hands are cleaned after toileting, before eating and at regular intervals throughout your shift. Being very busy is not an excuse for not ensuring a client's hygiene needs.

In this section you will learn about the **decontamination** techniques necessary to eliminate pathogens. Procedures for decontamination involve cleaning, disinfecting or sterilising.

> **decontaminate**
>
> *to make free from contaminants; this is done by cleaning, disinfecting or sterilising*

What you need to learn

- Objects and areas that are considered low risk in terms of being contaminated
- Objects and areas that are considered to be medium risk
- Objects and areas that are most definitely high risk

Outline the possible consequences of undergoing an operation in a room where objects and instruments are contaminated with pathogens.

Objects and areas that are considered low risk in terms of being contaminated

Areas considered low risk in terms of contaminants include floors, furniture and mobility aids. Cleaning such areas and equipment can be carried out using warm water and a good detergent.

Cleaning low-risk areas

Objects

Objects that are touched quite frequently might be washed or wiped down daily. After washing objects with detergent, a rinse may be necessary before objects are dried, preferably with paper towels or a disposable cloth.

Floors

Hard floors may be washed daily in care organisations, and although unlikely to be touched by hands, there is a possibility that clients will go on hands and knees on the floor and that workers may touch the floor, when emptying catheter bags for example. They are generally considered to be low risk. Floor mops should be cleaned in hot soapy water, rinsed, then wrung out and stored with the mop upside down, so that it dries.

Carpets should be vacuumed daily and shampooed and thoroughly cleaned about once every 6–8 months (cleaning schedules will have to plan for this). Carpeting can soon look dirty and shabby, which will not reflect a high standard of cleanliness. If possible, carpets are best avoided, however many people have them at home, where you might be working.

Objects and areas that are considered to be medium risk

Medium-risk objects are those that could be contaminated, for example toilet seats, toilet handles and toilet doors. Areas for food preparation and serving are also of medium risk, especially when dealing with raw food and cooked food in the same area.

Activities that involve medium-risk objects are consequently more risky than cleaning floors, for example giving a client a bedpan and taking it away after use. In this instance, gloves should always be used since the bedpan will contain urine and possibly faeces. If left on the side in the sluice area this will be a source of contamination. (Bedpans and urinals are often disposable and broken down in special macerators, but some will need to be washed in the bedpan washer or in the case of being in someone's home, washed and then disinfected). Wearing gloves is essential in this procedure followed by careful disposal, hand-washing and applying alcohol rub. Take great care in ensuring that contact surfaces such as door handles are also disinfected regularly.

Disinfection of medium-risk areas

Cleaning alone is insufficient for medium-risk areas and you need to ensure that disinfection takes place. Disinfection is a process that reduces the possibility of infection but does not totally eradicate it. It is achieved by heat (82 degrees Celsius for at least five minutes) or by chemicals, which are usually diluted in water. Alcohol wipes may be used on some areas where tainting will not be a problem. (Tainting means that a residue, such as a smell or taste, may be left behind so these products are not used where they may come into contact with food, for example on chopping boards and knives.)

Objects and areas that are most definitely high risk

Objects and areas considered high risk are those where the chances of contamination are high. An operating theatre is a prime example. If pathogens enter an open wound in this environment the individual's recovery from the operation will be made difficult. This is especially so because people who are ill, or recovering from major surgery, are very vulnerable to infection. Theatre staff must only work in their designated area, i.e. in the sterile (theatre) or the non-sterile (the pre-operative area or the recovery area) to reduce transport of pathogens.

Sterilisation of high-risk areas

The only acceptable method in this environment is sterilisation. This process makes objects pathogen-free and as such is the most suitable process for high-risk areas. It can be achieved by one of the following three methods:

- *Heat* – using high steam pressure (called autoclaving). Autoclaving is a process of high-heat steam (at 134 degrees Celsius) applied for about three minutes, and is suitable for instruments made of metal, for example surgical instruments. Boiling takes longer than high-pressure steam and is therefore not used as much.

- *Radiation* – this is the use of gamma rays (high-energy rays given off by some radioactive substances) to sterilise objects. Radiation is sometimes used to make food products safe, however this is not a process used on healthcare premises.

- *Chemicals* – sterilisation in chemical solutions is used for plastic materials which may melt under high-heat pressure, for example plastic utensils and babies' bottles and soothers.

Disinfection must follow thorough cleaning. It is not a stand-alone process. Instructions must be carefully followed and the disinfectant rinsed away before the area is dried. Storage of disinfectants must be away from other products and hands must be washed thoroughly after use. Again, you need to carefully follow the care setting's schedule for the patterns and frequency of disinfection. Infection control teams determine which products should be used in what areas and how to use these, for example how often and for what purpose.

Activity 30

Below is a list of objects you may encounter in a health or care setting. Tick to indicate whether the risk of contamination from each of these is low, medium or high.

Object	Low risk	Medium risk	High risk
1. Wooden floor			
2. Surgical scissors			
3. Urinal			
4. Window blind			
5. Shared books			
6. Toilet seats			
7. Door handles			
8. Food trolleys			
9. Mattress			
10. Chopping board for raw meat			

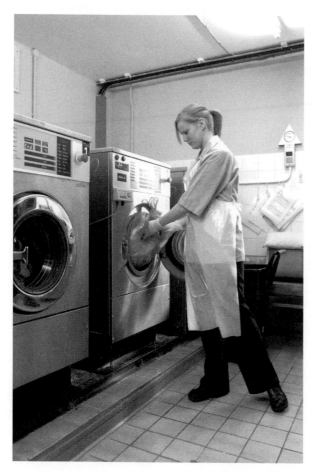

Cleanliness and order in all areas is essential to prevent the spread of infection.

3

Legislation relevant to infection prevention and control

3.1 Understand the legislation, regulations and guidance that govern infection prevention and control

It is important to be clear about the laws (legislation and regulations) you must follow in the workplace. Failure to follow these in your working practice may result in you being prosecuted (charged in a court of law).

Under current legislation, people who cause ill health to others will be fined heavily or sent to prison.

Laws are introduced for the safety of individuals, visitors, staff and the healthcare setting as a whole. The infection control teams and managers create policies that should clearly show how staff must act in order to follow current laws. Inspections are regularly carried out to ensure policies are adhered to. The Commission for Social Care Inspection (CSCI) is an organisation that has a duty to inspect care homes. The Healthcare Commission carries out checks of hospitals.

What you need to learn and be aware of

- Health and Safety at Work Act (1974)
- Management of Health and Safety at Work Act (amended 1999 to include risk assessing)
- Control of Substances Hazardous to Health (COSHH) Regulations (2002)
- Reporting of Injuries, Diseases and Dangerous Occurrences Regulations (RIDDOR) (1995)
- The Public Health (Control of Diseases) Act (1984)
- The Public Health (Infectious Diseases) Regulations (1988)
- Food Safety Act (1990)
- The Food Safety (General Food Hygiene) Regulations (Department of Health 1995)
- The Environment Protection (Duty of Care) Regulations (1991)
- Health Protection Agency Act (2004)
- Hazardous Waste Regulations (2005)
- NICE (National Institute for Health and Clinical Excellence) Guideline 2 (June 2003)

The Health and Safety at Work Act (1974)

This Act is the main piece of legislation regarding health and safety in the workplace. It places responsibilities on both employers and employees, who are jointly responsible for protecting the health and safety of all people using the workplace, whether staff, individuals or visitors. It is also concerned with the prevention of accidents and infection control. Legislation such as the COSHH and RIDDOR regulations (see pages 66–68) are an extension of the Health and Safety at Work Act.

The diagrams below show the different responsibilities for employers and employees under the Health and Safety at Work Act.

Read your workplace's policy on health and safety, then list the things you do to show you understand your responsibilities.

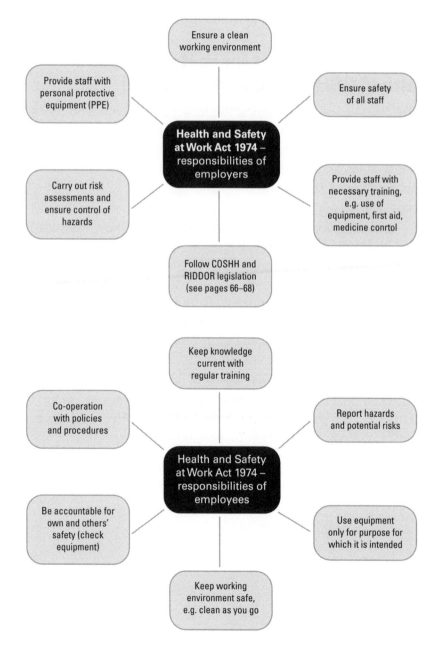

1. What risks might be posed in your workplace? How are these risks managed?

2. Why should you plan ahead to avoid risks and hazards?

The Management of Health and Safety at Work Act (amended 1999)

This Act introduced risk-assessing as a legal requirement for organisations. It requires both employers and employees to think about the risks involved in their work and to plan ahead to avoid these. These are the stages in this process:

- assess the risk to health and safety
- decide whether you can remove or reduce the risk
- if so, develop a workable plan to put this into practice
- having done this, review your actions so that you know it works, or try other measures to control the risk.

Risk assessment is discussed further in Unit 4.3.

The Control of Substances Hazardous to Health (COSHH) Regulations (2002)

COSHH regulations are intended to protect employees who come into contact with hazardous substances in the workplace. In health and social care settings, hazardous substances include cleaning materials, acids and disinfectants, as well as body products such as blood and urine.

COSHH regulations focus on how hazardous substances are used in the workplace, for example where they are kept, how they are labelled, their effects and how to deal with an emergency involving one. All hazardous substances should be stored in a safe place and containers must have safety lids and caps. They should also be clearly labelled, giving all necessary information about that substance, for example instructions on how to use the substance safely and what to do in the case of a spillage. Training is therefore essential.

A summary of the COSHH regulations is shown on page 67. Every workplace should have a member of staff who is responsible for implementing the guidelines set down by the COSHH regulations.

Understand the hazards, i.e. from cleaning fluids, waste, blood and urine

Store hazardous substances properly

COSHH regulations require you to...

Know how to deal with spillages and accidents involving hazardous substances

Understand labelling, expiry dates, instructions for use and warnings

1. Describe the actions that keep you and others safe when you are in contact with hazardous substances.

2. If you were unsure about which substances are considered hazardous or how to handle them, who would you go to for advice?

Activity 31

Describe in detail what should appear on labels on medications and cleaning fluids.

_____

_____

_____

_____

_____

_____

Who is responsible in your workplace for implementing the guidelines set down by the COSHH regulations?

Reporting of Injuries, Diseases and Dangerous Occurrences Regulations (RIDDOR) (1995)

RIDDOR makes the reporting and recording of injuries a legal requirement, in order to help with insurance claims and prevent accidents from recurring. All records of accidents must be available for inspection and kept for a period of three years.

Under RIDDOR, the following must be reported to the Health and Safety Executive:

- death or major injury, including referral to hospital and if visitors are involved
- any injury that results in an employee being off work for more than three days
- poisoning
- skin conditions such as dermatitis and skin cancer
- lung diseases including occupational asthma and those linked to asbestos
- occupational cancers
- musculo-skeletal disorders
- incidents including explosions, release of toxic gases or collapse of a lift.

In addition to reporting the above to the Health and Safety Executive, if you work with children you must also contact the Office for Standards in Education (OFSTED).

The Public Health (Control of Diseases) Act (1984)

This Act makes it a legal requirement for organisations to ensure that proper and adequate controls are in place for the safe disposal of waste, clean water and sanitation. The Act also deals with the control of certain diseases, notifiable diseases and immunisation. General practitioners must report suspected food poisoning or infections to the local environmental health officer or practitioner. The management of healthcare organisations, including hospitals and residential homes, should ensure that the cause of any infection is investigated fully.

The Public Health (Infectious Diseases) Regulations (1988)

This legislation states that data must be collected for certain infectious diseases in order that they can be monitored by the district health authority. This information would tell healthcare organisations of likely diseases in certain areas, the prevalence (number of incidences) of those diseases and possible vulnerable members of the public. Reports from the Health Protection Agency (see page 70) may give indications of how to control possible epidemics (mass outbreaks of those diseases). Should an outbreak of a notifiable disease occur, the act allows for vulnerable people to be immunised against the disease.

All the infectious diseases listed by this legislation are considered notifiable – that is, any occurrence of the disease should be reported to the appropriate authorities. However, the list of diseases is subject to change. For example, chickenpox used to be notifiable but this is no longer the case.

Food Safety Act (1990)

This Act ensures high standards for organisations serving and preparing food. It is illegal to provide food in an unfit-to-eat state. It should not be rotten, decomposing or contaminated. Those providing food to the public must be able to show that they have made every effort to ensure safety. Enforcement officers have the power to close premises and take legal action if standards have compromised food safety.

Another legal requirement of this Act is that food handlers who are infected (become ill with a disease) or are potential carriers (could pass a disease to others without becoming ill themselves) must stay away from work until all potential threats from transmission have been removed. The manager of premises must ensure that staff adhere to these requirements.

1. What diseases are currently notifiable?

2. Why do you think these diseases have been stated as notifiable?

Research an actual incident of food poisoning and trace the events that led to a resolution.

Activity 32

Two incidents of diarrhoea and vomiting have been reported among residents of a care home. Under the Food Safety Act, what should happen next?

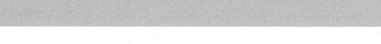

_____

_____

_____

_____

It is crucial for healthcare workers to maintain a very high standard of hygiene when handling food. With domiciliary care it is vital to educate the individual in effective hygiene measures for self-care procedures.

How do you dispose of the following?

1. Food waste

_____

_____

_____

2. Clinical waste, e.g. blood, urine, sharps, dressings, used intravenous catheters

_____

_____

_____

3. Recyclable material

_____

_____

_____

The Food Hygiene (England) Regulations (2006) and the Regulation (EC) 852/2004 on the hygiene of foodstuffs

These have replaced The Food Safety (General Food Hygiene) Regulations (Department of Health 1995). Almost all the requirements however are the same but the focus is on showing and *documenting* food safety management systems in accordance with what food is provided for the public. This is to ensure complete safety in provision.

These regulations are designed to ensure that food is stored, cooked and served in accordance with proper hygiene controls. It also gives powers to environmental health officers to manage inspections of organisations serving food and to respond quickly to reported outbreaks of food poisoning. The regulations apply to care homes and hospitals; however, it is difficult to investigate incidents in domiciliary care due to the independence of the individual.

The Environmental Protection (Duty of Care) Regulations (1991)

These regulations place a duty of care on all waste producers and those who manage waste, for example council-run refuse tips. Waste carriers must be registered with the Environment Agency. Producers of waste, for example care settings, must take responsibility for ensuring their waste is managed without harm to human health or the environment. The aim is to reduce fly tipping (dumping waste illegally) and waste crime. Organisations transferring waste are required to complete and retain a transfer note containing a written description of that waste.

The Health Protection Agency Act (2004)

This agency was started in April 2003 with the aim of reducing and controlling infectious diseases and biological hazards. It works in partnership with other health organisations, including those set up overseas, to prevent future outbreaks. The agency has regional and local teams throughout the country to recognise public health threats and bring a consistent unified approach to the management and prevention of infection. Meetings are held regularly to discuss what infections are happening and where. The agency also links with the NHS, particularly the regional primary care trusts and local government departments. The agency guides government policy and informs the public. At the time of print a big concern is the increase in sexually transmitted diseases in the UK.

The Hazardous Waste Regulations (2005)

Under these regulations, organisations disposing of hazardous waste (including medicines and yellow bags for incineration) need to register with the Environment Agency. If this is not done the waste will not be collected. In addition, any procedures in place for handling, treating, transporting and disposing of waste must be recorded and safety ensured to remove risks of contamination. The legislation also includes a list of hazardous waste products so that organisations can discuss correct procedures. In 2006, the Department of Health Environment Agency introduced a new European standard: 'The Safe Management of Healthcare Waste'. See the table below for details.

This colour-coded segregation system for the categorisation of waste has recently been introduced but continues to be under review in terms of the 'duty of care' requirements. It is by no means mandatory, but it is hoped that providers of healthcare will adopt a safe standardised process in line with waste-disposal requirements. The colour of the waste receptacle will determine on how the waste should be treated and disposed of.

The segregation of waste demands a risk assessment of each client's condition. Infectious waste must be placed in yellow bags, but orange bags labelled 'waste for alternative treatment' may also be suitable. Yellow-and-black bags are for offensive waste such as incontinence pads (if a client has diarrhoea, orange or yellow bags must be used). Check with management for the correct disposal procedure (managers should check with waste contractors). Fines can be imposed for faulty segregation of waste.

How does the work of the Health Protection Agency affect your work in the healthcare sector? To answer this question, carry out research using the agency's website. You can access this site by going to www.heinemann.co.uk/hotlinks, entering the express code 2323P and clicking on the relevant link.

What kind of infections and data do you think we ought to be informed about and why?

_____

_____

The new colour-coding system for hazardous clinical waste

Orange	Boxes or sacks for dressings, bandages and single-use plastic instruments; the bulk of community-care waste will be in orange receptacles
Yellow	Infectious waste for incineration only
Yellow/purple	Contents containing traces of cytotoxic drugs (used for chemotherapy), or anti-viral drugs
Yellow/black	Contents are neither infectious or hazardous
Black	Household waste

1. How do the Hazardous Waste Regulations affect your practice?

2. Why do you think the UK government wants healthcare settings to keep records of waste disposal?

Visit the website of NICE to find out more about the guidance available for healthcare settings and individuals, care workers and the general public. To access this site, go to www.heinemann. co.uk/hotlinks, enter the express code 2323P and click on the relevant link. You will also be able to order copies of NICE guidance via their website.

The NICE (National Institute for Health and Clinical Excellence) Guideline 2 (June 2003)

This organisation provides guidance on the promotion of good health and the prevention and treatment of ill health. This can be divided into three general areas:

- *public health* – those working in the NHS, local authorities and the wider public and voluntary sector
- *health technologies* – the use of new and existing medicines, treatments and procedures within the NHS
- *clinical practice* – appropriate treatment and care of people with specific diseases and conditions within the NHS.

NICE has provided guidance on infection control. This is available as two separate leaflets; one is for healthcare professionals and the other is for individuals, care workers and the general public. Topics include:

- ways of avoiding infection, including hand-washing
- the use of barrier aids, for example gloves and aprons
- using sharps safely
- general education about the principles of cross-infection.

Activity 33

Complete the table below by identifying the laws that the settings and care workers have broken.

1. The care home has no first aid box or workers trained in first aid	
2. The residential home for children has no records of risk assessments	
3. Staff have had no training on cleaning materials and use of disinfectants	
4. A staff member has sustained a needlestick injury but does not report this	

1. Name the agency responsible for monitoring infectious diseases in the UK.

2. What are the requirements of the Hazardous Waste Regulations 2005?

3. Name the organisation that produces publications for staff, individuals and visitors to increase awareness and education of infection control measures?

4. How can a healthcare setting ensure that all staff are aware of the requirements of legislation?

5. How is a suspected case of food poisoning managed?

6. List three notifiable diseases.

7. What does the Health Protection Agency do?

8. What is the role of environmental health practitioners?

9. What legislation states that it is illegal to serve food unfit for eating?

10. If you needed to be immunised against a disease, what legislation would provide for this?

1. Which legislation helps to control outbreaks of food poisoning?

_____

_____

2. Describe your actions under this legislation.

_____

_____

_____

_____

3.2 Understand the organisation's policies and procedures with regard to infection prevention and control

All healthcare sector organisations must follow legal requirements to maintain effective infection control. Working policies should be distributed to all staff, explaining how to work according to the law. The responsibility of the infection control teams ensures that up-to-date information is disseminated as and when it is needed.

It is your responsibility to follow your setting's working policies and be mindful of good practice at all times.

When you join a team, information, advice and guidance on following infection control procedures will be given as part of your induction. Some organisations will also arrange for external training, giving you the opportunity to gain an accredited award. This is a requirement of the Care Standards Act 2000.

Different organisations, different policies

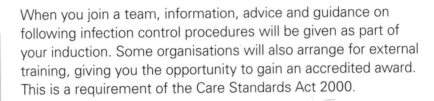

During the induction to infection control procedures in your setting, what things were highlighted as your specific duties to keep infection at bay?

Organisations delivering care differ in nature – some are large institutions while others involve caring for individuals in their own home or a small community setting. Working policies and procedures will differ accordingly. For example, it might not always be possible to witness the administering of medications in the person's own home.

You must be aware of your rights to personal safety when you work alone or when supporting a nurse working in the community. You must not travel alone at night or place yourself in a vulnerable position alone in a client's home. You must not attempt to work alone in any way if this threatens your personal or physical safety, for example lifting alone.

Information and guidance on good hygiene practice

Remember, under the Health and Safety at Work Act (see page 66), you have a right to be safe while performing your duties.

Posters and leaflets can be used to remind care workers, individuals and visitors of the need to adhere to good hygiene. Leaflets on hand-washing can be made freely available and posters and signs placed in appropriate locations to remind people to wash their hands.

The Royal College of Nursing has created an infection control checklist as part of its 'Wipe it Out' campaign to combat MRSA. To access this site, go to www.heinemann.co.uk/hotlinks, enter the express code 2323P and click on the relevant link.

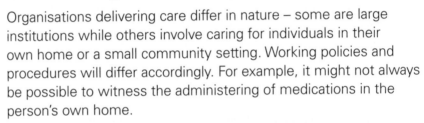

Activity 34

Carry out a check of your workplace to identify information and guidance on good hygiene practice. Are enough posters, leaflets and signs made available? If not, what opportunities are there for providing more?

_____

_____

_____

_____

1. Carry out research into the policies and procedures for infection control of the different care settings listed below.

   - community care
   - domiciliary care
   - hospital
   - nursing home
   - residential care.

2. Find out about how the policies in your workplace are monitored to ensure good infection control.

The National Institute for Health and Clinical Excellence (NICE) has produced a range of informative publications about preventing infection in care settings. These are targeted at nurses, care workers, visitors and workers linked to direct care. They are free of charge and have been distributed to GP surgeries, health centres, hospitals, care homes and residential homes.

1. How do you comply with PPE policy and practice in your working role?

2. If blood from an individual in your care splashed onto your face, what does your setting's policy say you must do?

3. What is a cleaning schedule?

4. What items need to be placed in yellow bags?

5. How do you advise members of the public when visiting potentially infectious clients?

4

Roles, responsibilities and boundaries

4.1 Understand the roles and responsibilities of personnel in relation to infection prevention and control

Each care worker must be responsible for their own actions at work with regard to protecting oneself and others from infection. It is irresponsible and unprofessional to disregard potential risks to health. If you became ill and had to be hospitalised, you would not want the staff who attended to you to be sloppy with regard to hygiene and care procedures. Similarly, you would not want your friends or relatives to receive anything less than the very best of care.

Many pathogenic organisms are easily transmitted between people, but infection will especially affect the very young, older people or those suffering from ill health. Policies to control infection have got to reach out to and involve everybody.

This section looks at the roles of various personnel (employees) within the health and social care sector. It should help you to understand the importance of all care workers, non-care workers, managers and specialist personnel complying with infection control.

Non-care workers are employed outside the immediate care environment but may influence infection control measures, for example gardeners, cooks, drivers and administration staff. Specialist personnel include infection control nurses and doctors, environmental health officers and staff of health protection units.

What you need to learn

- The role and responsibilities of care workers
- The role and responsibilities of non-care workers
- The role and responsibilities of managers
- The role and responsibilities of specialist personnel

The role and responsibilities of care workers

Care workers have a responsibility to themselves, their colleagues, the individuals in their care and visitors, to keep the risk of infection to an absolute minimum. This is achieved by the codes of conduct outlined below.

Codes of conduct for care workers

- Maintain good personal hygiene.
- Carry out thorough hand-washing before and after contact with individuals and in between tasks, after using the toilet and before handling food.
- Adhere to the rules of wearing clean protective clothing and equipment.
- Safely dispose of waste using the correct procedures, including disposal of sharps.
- Keep contact items clean and generally clean up as you go.
- Remain on your guard and report any potential hazards, including the behaviour of visitors.

It is worthwhile to stay abreast of any developments and current research. This will help you minimise risks of infection and make your job more interesting. It also provides possibility for career development.

The Care Standards Act 2000 and the Learning and Skills Council (LSC) made funds available for all care sector employees to gain a Level 2 qualification. This is often an NVQ (National Vocational Qualification) in Health and Social Care. The NVQ is based on national occupational standards of care and performances and is assessed chiefly in the workplace. Induction or foundation programmes should be completed within six weeks of commencement of employment.

Activity 35

Devise an information sheet for new staff to use in their induction period. It must state the ways in which staff members can reduce the risks of infection.

Activity 36

What would you say to these people if you discovered the following during a visit to their homes as a domiciliary care worker? How would you report these occurrences?

1. Tomas is leaving his soiled dressings on the kitchen work surface	
2. Samira has an 'itchy' rash on her arm	
3. Hilda is waiting until her incontinence pads are soaking wet before changing them	

Care scenario: Marie

Marie helps to change a soiled bed then carries the dirty sheets to the laundry skip down the corridor. As she walks, some of the sheets trail behind her on the floor. She is then asked to help Mrs Kaur with her lunch, which has just arrived. Marie quickly goes and cuts the sandwiches and pours Mrs Kaur a drink. Marie then has to empty Mrs Parry's urine catheter and leaves a specimen on the table in Mrs Parry's room.

List and explain how this healthcare assistant is not following good practice procedures.

_____

_____

_____

_____

The role of non-care workers in infection control may not initially appear important because of their lack of contact with vulnerable people. However, their working roles may easily impact on the health of those in your care.

The role and responsibilities of non-care workers

Non-care workers are those employed outside the immediate care environment. They can influence infection control measures through direct or indirect contact with the care environment and the individuals within it. Examples of non-care workers include gardeners, cooks, drivers, porters and administration staff.

Sometimes non-care workers will come into contact with individuals in care settings. If this happens, they will need to know from the care worker if there are any safety measures they should take, for example if the client is infectious.

What hazards does a driver who has a heavy cold pose to the many care homes he delivers to?

Care scenario: The gardener and the cook

Charles the gardener brings home-grown vegetables and flowers into the kitchen and places them on the work surface. Maria the cook is elsewhere so he leaves. Maria returns an hour later, in a hurry to prepare lunch. She moves the flowers and vegetables and prepares the chicken stew. She has washed the raw meat but the garden vegetables have been pushed against this on the work surface.

1. What potential hazards may have been introduced by the gardener and the cook?

   _____

   _____

   _____

2. Write what the gardener and the cook *should* have done to maintain control of infection.

   _____

   _____

   _____

In some organisations the administrations assistant has contact with individuals when taking their personal details before admission. It is therefore advisable that clerical staff in care settings are aware of the potential hazards and can report these following the admission procedure.

Cleaners have a responsibility to maintain the cleanliness of the buildings, especially in medium-risk areas such as toilets, bathrooms, kitchens and in high-risk areas such as operating theatres in hospital settings. Cleaners also need to be knowledgeable about micro-organisms and how diseases are spread. This is advisable for cleaners in any setting where care for vulnerable people takes place.

What advice would you give to non-care workers coming into your setting with regard to infection prevention and control?

People will work more effectively to prevent contamination if they appreciate the reasons for good practice.

The role and responsibilities of managers

The manager of any care sector organisation should be fully aware and knowledgeable about infection control policies and procedures, and the roles and responsibilities of all staff in terms of infection control.

Managers need to know about employees' skills, capabilities and knowledge base, so that an appropriate training and induction regime can be established. Managers need to continually check the performance of staff and support and guide them if there are any misunderstandings. This is regularly done by way of appraisals or supervision times.

As well as knowledge of their employees, managers should also know the condition of the individuals in their care. This is so that they can respond quickly to any signs of infection, for example by transferring an individual into a single room. Managers can arrange for nasal swabs to be taken, for example to confirm the presence of *Staphylococcus aureas*. If its presence is confirmed, they can arrange appropriate care.

Managers need to check the cleanliness of the rooms and the general environment on a regular basis. They should know who to contact when infections are suspected. This is usually the doctor or GP, but if necessary they will inform the public health department or the Health Protection Agency. They should ensure up-to-date knowledge of infection control and keep careful records of hygiene procedures such as regular cleaning and hand-washing.

Interview your manager to find out how policies and procedures regarding infection prevention and control are put into practice in your care setting. Document your findings.

Activity 37

Complete a table like the one below by giving an example of how a manager can perform the duties listed in the left-hand column.

Manager's role	How this can be performed
1. Know the knowledge and skills of staff	
2. Inform staff of policies and procedures to reduce infection risks	
3. Monitor ongoing performance of staff	
4. Respond to potential high-risk infection in individuals	
5. Prove that risks to infection have been removed or minimised	

The role and responsibilities of specialist personnel

Infection control nurses and doctors

These nurses and doctors work together in order to minimise infection in the community and in large public organisations such as hospitals. Their role is also to inform, educate and monitor procedures. They need to know when outbreaks occur, in order to investigate the causes and manage the solutions. They also work closely with government agencies so outbreaks do not occur again. Records are carefully stored in case others need to refer to them at a later stage.

Activity 38

Imagine that you are an infection control nurse. Tick the following issues if they concern you and state your immediate plan of action.

Issue	Concern? (✓)	Immediate action
1. Individual has diarrhoea and vomiting		
2. A wound is not healing		
3. Linen is regularly changed		
4. Updates on infection control are disseminated		
5. Mouse droppings are found in the food cupboard		

Environmental health officers

Environmental health officers, or practitioners, carry out various checks and investigations to ensure public health and safety. The areas of public health with which they are concerned include food safety, workplace health and safety policies, housing conditions, industrial waste, animal health, contaminated land and infectious diseases. They also:

- give advice on how to reduce and prevent the spread of infection and disease
- investigate reports into threats to public health, for example food poisoning, poor hygiene, and organisations and homes where waste is accumulating
- take samples for laboratory analysis
- take action to put in force laws like the Food Safety Act (see page 69) or the Hazardous Waste Regulations 2005 (see page 71)
- have a licence to enter and examine properties.

The work of health protection teams

People in health protection teams study the causes of outbreaks of infection and advise the government accordingly. For example, the Health Protection Agency (see page 70) is responsible for monitoring infectious diseases and patterns of illness. This involves looking at patterns of disease in other countries, since global travel creates the risk that these diseases could be brought back to the UK.

Activity 39

The table below lists different organisations and teams concerned with infection prevention and control. Complete the table by carrying out research into the role of each one.

Organisation	Role in infection prevention and control
1. Strategic Health Authorities	
2. Healthcare Commission	
3. Health and Safety Executive	
4. National Institute for Health and Clinical Excellence	
5. Infection Control Team	
6. Health Protection Units	

Health and safety policies and procedures are put in place to protect all care workers, clients, visitors and the care setting in general. It is important that everybody works together to achieve high standards in care sector organisations. Low standards in care homes will be reported to the Commission for Social Care Inspection, while low standards in hospitals will be reported to the Healthcare Commission. Should this occur, morale will fall among care workers and other staff, people may lose their jobs and settings will earn a poor reputation and may even have to close.

All organisations and care settings have a legal duty to ensure that workers are informed of health and safety policies and procedures. This includes any changes introduced by management or law. Sometimes procedures are short-term measures; for example, if structural work such as kitchen alterations is being carried out, alternative arrangements will need to be made regarding the preparation, serving and disposal of food to ensure high standards of infection control are maintained.

This section looks at a number of common policies and procedures that affect healthcare personnel and visitors.

You have a duty to protect the individuals in your care. Giving your very best will raise standards and make your work with others more rewarding.

What you need to learn

- Reporting of infectious or notifiable diseases and outbreaks
- Seeking advice and guidance
- Admissions, transfers and discharges of individuals
- Documentation and record keeping in relation to infection
- Following the death of an individual
- Handling, collection and storing of specimens
- Encourage all visitors to comply with hygiene policies and procedures

Which legislation states that employers are responsible for ensuring there is a written safety policy that is understood by all staff?

_____

_____

Reporting of infections or notifiable diseases and outbreaks

The Reporting of Injuries, Diseases and Dangerous Occurrences Regulations (RIDDOR) 1995 (see page 68) state that employees have a legal duty to inform the Health and Safety Executive or local authority environmental health department of the following in terms of infection:

- possible poisonings
- contagious diseases such as hepatitis, tuberculosis, Legionnaires' disease and tetanus
- acute illness that may be caused by workplace toxins or infected material.

Accident report forms

Workers involved with any of the above and/or accidents must complete an accident report form. This is a requirement by law. Every workplace should have an accident report form as correct recording of an accident, incident or near-miss is important. All records of accidents must be available for inspection by the Commission for Social Care Inspection (CSCI) and kept for a period of three years.

Accident report forms must not give personal details of those involved in the accident or incident. This is a requirement of the Data Protection Act 1998, which aims to ensure that only relevant information is collected about individuals and that personal information remains confidential and is stored in a secure place.

Find your setting's accident report form. List the information that needs to be recorded on the form.

_____

_____

_____

_____

_____

_____

Accident report forms may be used in a court of law, so attention to objective and accurate detail is essential.

Seeking advice and guidance

Following infection control policies may not always seem easy. If you are uncertain, just ask – remember, your line manager is there to support you. Workers and managers in care settings should also be able to contact individuals and organisations to help them with policy-making and to address any uncertainties. These might include, for example, the infection control team, the local health centre, NHS Direct (also gives useful website information) or the public and environmental health departments of the local authority and/or hospitals.

You can access a plethora of information, advice and guidance via the Internet; many websites contain guidance on good practice. Local authorities will also help with more local issues, for example, the day and time of refuse collections. Textbooks are easily accessible and regularly updated. The government website gives information on current legislation and reforms in terms of infection control.

Seeking further training

Managers of care settings are responsible for informing staff about their role and responsibilities with regard to infection control. New staff should complete their induction within six weeks of starting their job. Thereafter, managers have a responsibility to ensure that staff are informed of any changes to working policy. Care workers should complete training programmes to at least Level 2 and beyond if they wish to become managers themselves.

Regular training and updates maintains the professionalism of care workers. Individuals and visitors often ask care workers why procedures are in place. It would prove embarrassing if you couldn't explain this accurately and confidently, and individuals and visitors might lose respect for staff and the care setting.

Making complaints

If you wish to complain about unsatisfactory practice, this should be reported verbally to the line manager but also documented in detail (remember to protect the personal details of people implicated in the report). Guidance here should focus on positive measures to remove risks and improve hygiene and safety practices.

To access some websites containing guidance on good practice in relation to infection control, visit the Heinemann website at www.heinemann.co.uk/hotlinks, then enter the express code 2323P and click on the relevant links. Which websites are most useful to your work?

Infection control is very important and if there is any misunderstanding of issues you should be offered further training.

Admission, transfer and discharge of individuals

The admission, transfer and discharge of individuals each carries the risk of infection, so there needs to be guidance on these procedures to avoid cross-infection.

Admission

When an individual is referred to a residential home or hospital, some prior knowledge about his or her condition needs to be known so that staff can prepare equipment, space, materials, special diets and medication. Care plans will follow an initial examination that will identify any skin lesions and problems that may indicate the need for separation from others. In some instances items may be needed very quickly after admission, as for example when an individual needs to occupy a separate room and be nursed in isolation.

Sometimes equipment will come with individuals who are being admitted, and may be used solely for that individual. People admitted with possible infections should have nasal swabs (anterior nares), throat, skin, sputum or wound swabs taken for analysis of pathogenic micro-organisms. Isolation nursing may start immediately; results from nasal swabs can be obtained within 24 hours.

Transfer

As with admission, if an individual needs to be transferred to another room or ward it is essential that any new staff looking after this person have the right information. The client also will need support in adjusting to a new environment. Equipment and materials may follow the client to a new room, but toilet facilities and new routines will need to be sensitively explained.

After the individual leaves the ward or room, staff must clean the bed and mattress thoroughly, disinfect objects in the room, including fittings, and then apply clean sheets to the bed. It is a good idea to throw open windows to allow the circulation of fresh air, if possible.

Discharge of individuals

When the time comes for individuals to be discharged it is crucial to give them any information that they may need in order to keep themselves and others free from infection. This might simply be a reminder of good hygiene techniques, particularly if the individual is being discharged with a wound. Any other agencies, e.g. community nurses and carers, should be informed of the care routine established.

Individuals should also be supplied with:

- an adequate supply of sterile dressings (these may be provided by a community nurse)
- if using sharps, the proper containers and details of how to obtain supplies
- instructions about safe disposal of waste or soiled materials. This may involve the collection of soiled and/or used dressings in the appropriate yellow bags.

If the individual has:

- a feeding tube into the stomach
- a central venous catheter
- a urinary catheter
- a colostomy

then detailed instructions should be given on how to care for these to avoid infection. This includes effective hand-washing techniques using soap and water, followed by alcohol hand-rubs. (For further information on indwelling catheters and enteral feeding, see pages 93–94.)

Documentation and record-keeping in relation to infection

In hospitals, care homes and domiciliary care, documentation is essential to ensuring quality of provision. It also provides clear evidence for inspectors of care settings that processes and procedures are being carried out properly. Inspections assess the direct care of individuals as well as environmental risks and management of food safety.

Direct care of individuals

From admissions, the specific care of the individual is documented to include:

- how that person needs help
- the medications he or she is taking
- his or her preferred diet
- any special requirements for treatments, for example care of a urinary catheter, enteric feeding tube or colostomy.

Once documented in a care plan, the actual treatments are confirmed by dates, times and signatures. This is so that staff are aware of when treatments took place. Some records require comments, such as records of examinations of wounds. If a wound looks sore and red, or there is a discharge, this needs to

The National Institute for Health and Clinical Excellence (NICE) has produced leaflets to help individuals with these procedures. These are free of charge, and you will be able to order copies via their website. To access the site, go to www.heinemann. co.uk/hotlinks, enter the express code 2323P and click on the relevant link.

How do you document the care of individuals in your setting? Give examples of the information you write down and how it is recorded.

Everyone working within any care setting needs to ensure good hygiene. Any areas that look dirty must be reported and spillages quickly and efficiently cleaned up. There is always a complaints procedure and this may involve staff, individuals or visitors making a written complaint in terms of observed poor hygiene.

With reference to what you have learned so far, what do you think food management documentation will record? It might help you to reflect on HACCP (hazard analysis critical control point) which identifies potential risks involved in the process of receiving raw food through to cooking and serving.

be documented and any treatment given clearly stated. Again, it is essential to state the date and time, and to provide a signature. Wound dressings and supplies may need to be accounted for and more supplies ordered. It is essential to maintain sterility so dressings need to be readily available. Care staff need to record their actual duties for each shift, which may include informing the individual and any visitors of personal hygiene requirements.

Care of the environment

Cleaning staff should maintain records of when and how they clean rooms, corridors, toilets and reception areas. They also need to report when cleaning materials and substances such as detergents and disinfectants are low. This also serves as evidence to line managers that good cleaning is being carried out because the substances are being used.

Infection incidents

responsible organisms

pathogenic micro-organisms that cause disease

Other records will include the number of reported cases of infection and the **responsible organisms** once identified by the laboratories. Accident and incident reports will reveal the number of needlestick injuries or spillages of contaminated fluids. Records must also show the results of these incidents, for example whether the affected person was referred to occupational health and if blood samples were taken. Dates and signatures should always be clear. It will also be necessary to include the date and time the incident was reported to the health and safety executive, and any advice given by them.

Audits

audit

a checking process to ensure standards are maintained

An **audit** is a checking process that is carried out by an internal person (for example an infection control nurse) and sometimes involving an external body. The external body for social care is the Commission for Social Care Inspection (CSCI). The Healthcare Commission carries out audits on hospitals, to ensure good individual care and that hospital management systems are maintained to a high standard.

Audits are necessary to ensure that healthcare personnel receive training, are able to carry out their duties and that procedures are being performed properly. Records of audits should be made available to inspectors of care settings or hospitals.

Activity 40

The table below lists the standard principles for auditing high standards of infection control as stated in NICE Clinical Guideline 2 (June 2003). Assess your own organisation by using the Yes and No columns. If you have ticked the 'No' column, what might be the appropriate action in each case?

Criterion	Method of data collection	Yes (✓)	No (✓) / Actions?
1. All healthcare personnel have an appropriate supply of hand decontamination equipment, gloves, aprons and protective clothing in their setting	Self-audit		
2. All healthcare personnel involved in care are trained and updated	Review of staff education records		
3. All individuals and care workers are aware of the need to: a) decontaminate hands b) use protective clothing c) dispose of sharps safely	Direct questioning of individuals and care workers		

Following the death of an individual

Upon the death of an infected individual, protective procedures to eliminate infections are vital. During the procedure of **last offices**, staff will need to wear aprons, masks and disposable gloves. Care should be taken with body fluids, for example discharges and urine, including in catheters. All dressings and appliances must be placed in a red bag or similar and marked with a hazardous waste label. The body will be transferred to the **mortuary** in a container bag marked 'infectious'.

After the body has been removed, the room must be cleaned and disinfected, windows opened and internal furniture and furnishings cleaned and disinfected.

last offices
the final care duty carried out for a person who has died. It involves bathing the person and dressing him or her in a clean gown, avoiding the spillage of body fluids.

mortuary
place where dead bodies are kept before burial or cremation

Handling, collection and storing of specimens

Under which legislation are deaths reported?

_____

Discharges from the body are high risk for being contaminated.

The types of specimens collected in a care environment include urine, sputum, pus from a wound, a throat swab, a nasal swab, vomit and faeces. Collecting samples involves a non-touch technique (i.e. using disposable gloves). The transferral to the lab is non-touch and, once in the lab, staff will examine the samples without touching them or breathing them in, as samples may give off airborne microbes. Each sample container is always carefully labelled to indicate what it holds and the individual's name. Jar lids must be secure and bags sealed. Training is needed for those who collect, transfer, transport or handle specimens or healthcare waste.

If samples cannot be transported to the lab straight away they must be stored in a fridge. However, the fridge must be used for specimens only and must not contain food. The low temperature of the fridge helps prevent the growth of pathogens and ensures that the sample indicates the actual pathogen on the individual and not one grown in poor storage conditions.

Encourage all visitors to comply with hygiene policies and procedures

Visitors to care establishments are welcome because family and friends help individuals on the road to recovery. However, they do pose a risk in terms of infection control. Visitors will sit on beds and touch clients without washing their hands, and in this way could pass on pathogens. If visitors do remember to wash their hands, is this done efficiently? Does the care establishment provide sufficient facilities to enable visitors to do this?

Residential homes and homes for the learning disabled or young people

People need to feel comfortable in the home where they live, so if you care and support people in their homes you should respect their routines and belongings. You do, however, have to work by your code of practice in maintaining consistently high standards of hygiene, and be aware of potential hazards that will alert you to a risk in limiting infection.

Care scenario: Amelia

Amelia has had diarrhoea for two days. The doctor has requested a sample to be sent to the lab.

Describe the procedure you need to follow in getting hold of the specimen and arranging for its transfer to the lab. Include details of what needs to be recorded.

Polite reminders to residents may have to be repeated, but this is part of your role as a carer: being patient and sensitive to people's needs. Once you have read this book all the signs that indicate a risk and a hazard will be easy for you, and you will know exactly what needs to be done.

Informing visitors of hygiene procedures

To ensure that visitors to care settings are aware of the importance of following hygiene procedures, they must be given the correct information. NICE provides publications for the promotion of good hygiene (see also pages 72 and 75). Some care settings also produce their own leaflets or display posters. It is better to be positive about good hygiene than to promote a fear-orientated environment, wherever you work in care.

Care scenario: Advising the visitor

You notice a gentleman visitor sitting on frail Mr Yassef's bed. He has brought him some snacks and now starts to feed Mr Yassef. You have not observed the visitor washing his hands.

How would you approach this situation?

1. Why do hospitals, nursing and residential homes need policies and procedures for infection control?

2. Why should any worker seek guidance on policies and procedures for infection control?

3. What specimens may be needed to identify possible causes of infections?

4. Why are specimens awaiting collection kept in a fridge?

5. If an individual has to be transferred to another room, what safety measures are necessary to minimise the risks of infection?

6. Why are visitors a potential hazard in terms of minimising infections?

7. List three duties of an infection control nurse.

8. What does HACCP mean?

9. What is the role of the Healthcare Commission?

10. What does NICE stand for and what does it do?

The Management of Health and Safety at Work Act (see page 66) made it a legal requirement that risk assessments are carried out in the workplace. This section will help you to know and understand the stages involved in the practice of risk assessment.

What you need to learn

- Identification of hazards
- Assessing the risks
- Recording the risks
- Removing/reducing the risks
- Reviewing the risks regularly

A hazard is anything that has the potential to cause harm. Risk is the likelihood of that hazard causing harm. For example, hazards in terms of infection control are pathogens. Some pathogens are considered a greater risk than others, for example MRSA or *Clostridium difficile*.

Identification of hazards

Hazards in care settings with regard to infection prevention and control are pathogens and anything that could support their growth and transmission. Because pathogens flourish only in certain environmental conditions it follows that to help prevent and control infection we need to ensure the environment does not support their growth. Thus possible breeding grounds for pathogens need to be identified.

Because pathogens can be spread from person to person, it follows that all people in a care setting are potentially hazardous. It is therefore important for people to minimise any behaviours that help pathogens to spread.

1. With reference to what you have learnt so far, list the causes of the growth of pathogens. (Refer to page 36 if you get stuck.)

2. Now list potential breeding grounds for pathogens in a care setting.

The structure and organisation of the care setting

The way in which buildings are structured and organised can create opportunities for pathogens to grow and spread. Hazards in this sense include, for example:

- There may be very few single rooms in which infections can be contained.
- Toilets and bathrooms may be communal so used frequently by potentially infected individuals and/or those who are weak and vulnerable.
- There may be too few wash basins or they may be badly placed. They may be without a plentiful supply of liquid soap, paper towels and waste bins.

- Kitchens may be badly situated, for example meals may have to be wheeled past toilets, sluices and waste areas.
- Kitchens may be old with evidence of peeling paint and damp surfaces where pathogens may lurk.
- Bed spaces may be overcrowded, making it easier for airborne microbes to infect neighbouring individuals.
- Certain routines may pose a hazard. For example, if food is arriving and beds are being stripped and changed, microbes can become airborne and contaminate food. This should definitely be avoided.

People who use the care setting

All people who use the care setting have the potential to spread pathogens. The likelihood of this occurring will vary for different people, for example clients, care workers, non-care workers or visitors. For each group you will need to consider the ways in which they might spread infection to others or become contaminated. This might include, for example:

- how much contact they have with different people in the care setting
- the areas of the building they use and the objects they come into contact with
- how much they know about infection control and hygiene procedures.

It is essential to consider whether the individuals in your care are reasonably fit, mobile and independent. They have choices and rights to make their own decisions about how they are cared for. It is your duty as their carer to modify risky behaviour and to enable them to make informed decisions about care that involves a shared pattern of responsibility for good hygiene.

Do they need invasive treatments such as catheterisations or central venous pressure lines for medicines to be given?

Indwelling catheters

If someone has an indwelling catheter it is important to advise them to inform you of any irritations or a frequent urge to pass urine and only passing small amounts. The catheter may become blocked and you will need to observe for this and any presence of blood or discharge in the tube. Routine cleaning of the area where the catheter enters the body is essential, but also to ensure careful drying and disposal of the tissue or towel used.

With reference to what you have learnt so far, list the different ways in which people can help pathogens to spread. (Refer to pages 38–9 if you get stuck.)

The catheter valve should remain closed unless needing to empty the bag and the bag should be below the bladder to allow good drainage. You should check that bags never touch the floor, either when the client is in bed or mobile.

Enteral feeding

This is the process of giving liquid feeds via a tube that can be:

- directly into the stomach (gastrostomy)
- naso-gastric (a tube via the nose to the stomach)
- directly into the small bowel (jejunostomy).

Before administering a feed it is important to:

- wash hands thoroughly
- use pre-packaged feed and note that the date has not expired and that storage was suitable according to instructions
- do not touch the feed and use clean equipment
- use cooled boiled water for mixing purposes
- flush the tube with the cooled water before and after the feed
- dispose of the packaging and administration sets immediately as household waste.

Those who are weakened by illness or lack of function are considered a bigger threat in terms of infection control. Giving high standards of care means that you are protecting them from contamination and playing a vital role in the prevention and control of infection.

Staff working in a care setting will also create their own hazards, for example depending on whether they are experienced or new to the role. In this instance, both groups could be identified as a potential hazard: the first group may become complacent through familiarity with the routines, and the second group may have little or no knowledge of how infections are minimised and require training. This highlights the importance of all staff being regularly reminded about hygiene and infection control measures.

List the ways in which individuals who are weakened by illness, surgery or lack of function can be considered a hazard in terms of infection control.

List the ways in which non-care workers might spread infection to others.

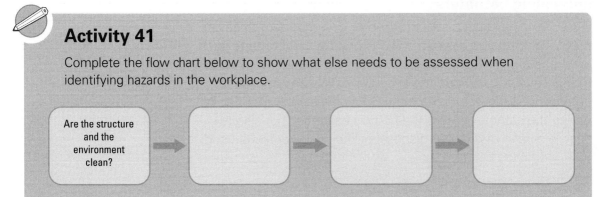

Activity 41

Complete the flow chart below to show what else needs to be assessed when identifying hazards in the workplace.

Are the structure and the environment clean? →   →   →

Assessing the risks

Once hazards in the care setting have been identified it is necessary to assess the risks each one poses. In other words, what potential does each hazard have to cause harm?

Risk assessments aim to identify hazards within building structures and practices in order to determine what steps can be taken to remove or minimise them. The table below lists different hazards that have the potential to cause infection. The risk assessments concerning them identify the nature of the risk and the actions required to deal with the hazard. A risk rating of high, medium or low is also given. Hazards with a high risk rating require more urgent attention (are considered a higher priority).

Hazard	Risk assessment	Risk rating
Flow of work duties	Waste and its disposal often come into contact with food production and serving; risk of cross-contamination unless new procedures are introduced	High
Peeling paint and cracked tiles	Likely to contain pathogens so needs repairing/replacing	Medium
Communal toilet areas	More regular cleaning needed to ensure cleanliness and prevent cross-contamination; also to ensure supplies of soap and paper towels are maintained	Medium
Air quality on hospital wards	Wards often feel 'stuffy'; risk of stale air and fumes. Routine window-opening needed to circulate fresh air	Low
Position of beds on hospital wards	In some wards beds are too close together, increasing risk of cross-infection	Medium
Facilities for isolation nursing	Only two isolation rooms available per ward and more needed. Arrangements need to be made to relocate individuals requiring isolation to another setting	High
Training for staff on safe practice procedures	Training updates required for experienced staff on hygiene, infection prevention and control	Medium
Residents in a home for the learning disabled display poor hygiene habits	Lack of awareness and understanding of hazards in the quest for independent living. Requires sensitivity to needs and education in ways to support independent living	Medium
Washing machine broken in client's own home; client often incontinent	How to launder bed sheets while the washing machine is being repaired: consult specialist incontinence nurse	Medium

Activity 42

Complete the table below by identifying four hazards in the illustration and their associated risks.

Hazard	Risk
1.	
2.	
3.	
4.	
5.	

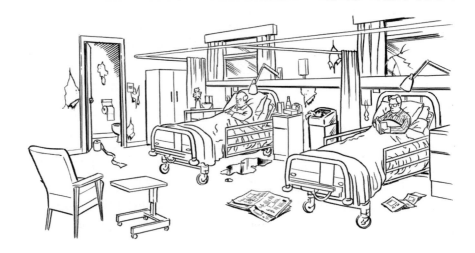

Recording the risks

If risks and hazards are not recorded, it may be difficult to make improvements to an establishment's structure or routine practices. Changes involving funding from outside agencies need to be backed up by evidence, such as signed reports. This evidence must show that money is being spent in the right places and not wasted.

A second factor for recording hazards and risks relates to legal requirements. It is a legal requirement by the Management of Health and Safety at Work Act (see page 66) that risk assessments are carried out and any issues reported. Employees are seen as responsible for their actions, and it may be necessary to make statements in a court of law. Records of incidents involving food will help to identify the cause of an outbreak of food poisoning. This process of record-keeping is a legal requirement by the Reporting of Injuries, Diseases and Dangerous Occurrences Regulations (RIDDOR) (see page 68).

> **How are risks reported and recorded in your workplace?**

Care scenario: Keeping good records

The chef of a residential home is summoned to court following a serious food poisoning outbreak.

To show good hygiene and food-safety practice, what records will the chef need to prove he keeps?

Removing or reducing the risks

Based on a risk assessment, plans will be made to either remove the hazards completely or reduce their effects. However, in practice, ideal conditions are not always possible. For example, we cannot wait for new buildings if we are looking after people in old ones – we just have to do the very best we can. Fortunately in hospitals, old structures such as 'nightingale' wards (long halls in which beds are placed in rows down each side of the room) are now much fewer. Care and residential homes now by law contain en-suite facilities.

Should individuals need isolation care and there are no single-room facilities, space must be given to allow the bed area to be well apart from other people. Any nursing care should be limited to one care worker only per shift. Visitors need to wear gowns and gloves that are disposed of at the end of the visit.

Regarding poorly assessed practices, such as inappropriately timed routines, changes can be more easily implemented.

- Bed baths and changes in the morning should be carried out before applying dressings; ideally, dressings should be applied in a clean room.
- Lunch should be scheduled to be served after all risk procedures are completed.
- If wash basins are too few in number, alcohol gels should be freely available, in containers or attached to uniforms.
- All staff should receive regular training on infection control measures. Dates of attendance should also be recorded.
- Residents in care homes should all have their clothing labelled and washed separately if any sign of contamination is noticed.

Posters and leaflets should be clearly displayed in establishments and should get the message across strongly about good hygiene and proper hand-washing techniques. These can be in toilets and bathrooms, and positioned on walls outside individuals' rooms. Posters can also remind visitors not to visit if they have a cough and/or cold.

Review the risks regularly

How do you know if measures to minimise infections are working?

In order to check whether measures to reduce risks are working, they need to be closely monitored and practices evaluated.

As a care worker, professionalism requires a high standard of care delivered consistently in a clean and hygienic environment. To this end, your working practices should be regularly monitored and reviewed. Any changes to improve practice should be made as soon as possible. You also need to be aware of any knowledge updates and research findings. Finally, you need to be on your guard about the risky behaviours of others and take steps to stop or reduce them.

By the terms of the Health and Safety at Work Act (1974), you are liable for your actions and omissions (failure to act) regarding your responsibilities to others. The individuals in your care depend on you for high-quality care – that is, the care you would like to receive if you were ill! Individual care means that practice is tailored to specific needs, with those with low immunity receiving the highest level of protection that is never compromised.

1. Why is the management of identified hazards and risks important?

2. Why does the management of identified hazards and risks need to be an ongoing exercise in the healthcare sector?

3. Give an example of a pathogen that is currently a cause for concern in healthcare settings and explain why this is.

4. List the possible hazards in an old building in terms of minimising the risk of infection.

5. How might visitors and non-care workers pose a threat to infection control?

6. Why do you think both experienced and new staff need regular updating on infection control?

7. How would you assess too few wash basins: low, medium or high risk?

8. What Act of Parliament would a care setting have broken if no risk assessments are recorded?

Trainer notes

The following teaching notes are intended to guide delivery of the Knowledge set for infection prevention and control and to provide a useful source of information for both tutors and learners. Answers are provided to all the Activities and Care scenarios, but learners should be advised to find their own answers before checking their accuracy using this section. Further teaching notes are given on some of the Look it up and Reflection features. There are also ideas for how to extend activities where relevant, including mention of how activities might be developed to suit different learning styles (visual, audio and kinaesthetic).

Before commencing a training programme on infection control it is advisable to ascertain the level of knowledge and experience that learners bring with them. This can be achieved by simply asking questions or using a short quiz as an icebreaker. The responses should provide a base on which to build the programme.

Icebreakers

Icebreaker quizzes can be visual, auditory or involve movement, which is a kinaesthetic approach.

- *Visual* might be the use of pictures for learners (in groups) to identify.
- *Auditory* might be listening to the tutor describing bacteria or an infection.
- *Kinaesthetic* could involve learners moving around the room doing activities such as investigating bacteria (with the use of a microscope, for example).

The icebreaker should only be a short warm-up exercise with the intention of inspiring learners to want to know more. It will also help them get to know one another. A more fun scenario is role-play; for example learners could be given cards stating whether they are a bacterium, antibody or antibiotic and asked to present a 5-minute play.

Introduce boundaries

Learners need simple rules to abide by and ones they are reminded of constantly, if necessary. Simplicity is more likely to be met with compliance and here are a few suggestions:

- good timekeeping
- adhere to rules of confidentiality in terms of anything a learner discloses (the exception is where an individual may be at risk)
- make connections of knowledge to own practice
- reflect on outcomes in own practice as a result of knowledge gained
- agree to listen to comments and never to interrupt
- challenge any statements you disagree with, but not the person who makes them.

1. Cause and spread of infection

1.1 Understand the definition of infection and colonisation

This section focuses on general systemic infection, localised infection and harmless colonisation of normal flora. The most important learning objective is for learners to recognise the differences between them in order to respond appropriately. As an introductory session on infection, learners could carry out one of the following activities:

- *Learners' style – audio:* learners could explore their own definitions of: infection, colonisation, pathogenic microbes, bacteria, toxins, systemic, localised, signs and symptoms. This could be a split exercise (perhaps in pairs).

- *Learners' style – visual:* learners could examine photos of systemic infections and localised infections, bacteria and toxins.
- *Learners' style – kinaesthetic:* definitions can be pre-set and arranged on cards in various places in the classroom. Learners can locate and match the definitions.

Activity 1

Learners are asked to recall any systemic infection they have experienced. Encourage them to focus on descriptions and feelings. Record their feedback on a flip chart.

Activity 2

Learners complete a table for different systemic infections, working in pairs or small groups. This activity is to reinforce recognition that diseases affect different body parts and yield different signs and symptoms. They can research the diseases listed on pages 4–5 or suggest alternatives.

Learner's style – visual: to extend this exercise, learners could collect or photocopy pictures of the infections. They could then design information leaflets on one or more of the systemic infections they have researched.

Care scenario: Harry

1. Harry has a localised infection.
2. The entry of pathogens via the cut may cause a localised inflammatory response.

Further questioning may prompt learners to think of how localised infections become systemic infections.

To extend learners' understanding of localised infections, you could organise them into three groups to carry out research into abscess formation, bites and stings, or cuts and grazes. Visual learners can collect pictures or illustrate their research; kinaesthetic learners can 'plot' the story of a localised infection along a wall frieze; audio learners might report their findings verbally.

Activity 3

Learners should answer these questions working on their own.

1. Learners identify three signs of infection. Answers could include rashes, flushed face, high temperature, oozing wound or pus, vomiting, diarrhoea.
2. Learners describe three complaints that may indicate that an individual has an infection. Answers could include headache, feeling hot, loss of appetite, nausea, lethargy, aching limbs.

Care scenario: Laura

1. Laura may have caught an infection while on holiday abroad.
2. Although Laura has recovered from the illness, she may still be a carrier and could pass the pathogen on to others.

3. Laura has recovered from her illness but more vulnerable people, such as the very young, older people or the immuno-suppressed, may be severely affected by it.

Learners should explore the possible consequences of contracting an illness in another country. Issues raised should include:

- the prevalence of disease in other countries
- the implications of being a carrier in the UK
- how colonisation may not cause disease.

Activity 4: De-colonisation

Learners might be encouraged to think of routines in the workplace in order to put this in perspective. They might like to interview others and do a general survey, and even compile results in a graph format. These suggestions would support all learning styles.

Pathogenic organisms can colonise via . . .	I can help to stop this by . . .
Coughing and sneezing	Not coming to work if ill Encouraging clients to use disposable tissues Washing hands after coughing and sneezing into tissues or hands Discouraging any sharing of objects Discouraging visitors who may be ill Wearing disposable gowns, gloves and masks
Blood and body fluids	Wearing disposable gloves when disposing of soiled articles or linen Ensuring correct disposal procedure Washing hands with liquid soap, warm water and using alcohol rub Wearing disposable gloves when changing catheter bags or dealing with enteric feeding tubes Qualified staff using aseptic techniques when catheterising and ensuring sterile needles when administering injections Wearing disposable aprons Changing uniform if it becomes contaminated during a shift Immediately cleaning up after spillages and disinfecting contaminated areas
Direct contact	Keeping bed area and table surfaces clean Regularly cleaning and disinfecting sluice area, toilets and bathrooms Washing hands after every potentially harmful procedure and between clients Washing hands before dealing with food Ensuring rapid and correct disposal of all waste items
Ingestion	Ensuring food is stored, cooked and served hygienically Ensuring clients' and own hands are washed before serving/eating

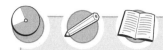

Activity 5

Learners create mind-maps for three key terms from this section. They may work in pairs or small groups to complete them. Some learners may experience difficulty in completing all the arrows and may require help. Time should be given to carrying out research and gathering materials before completing the mind-map.

with the different mechanisms to fight infection. Once completed, each group could explain how the mechanisms work in a feedback presentation. Challenge learners as to the circumstances that might reduce the effect of the mechanisms and why (illness; immaturity of the system; the immune system being suppressed; damage and trauma to tissues; general stress and weakening of the system in the elderly).

1.2 Understand how micro-organisms cause infection

Care scenario: Dennis

1. Dennis not washing his hands properly may result in an outbreak of food poisoning.

2. The consequences for the hospital if there was an outbreak of food poisoning include: exposure in the media; low morale of staff; poor reputation of the organisation; possibly lack of funding in future.

This Care scenario can be extended using the Look it up activity on page 73, which asks learners to research laws that deal with food poisoning.

the Look it up activity on page 73

Activity 6

Learners complete a spider diagram to summarise their understanding of how the body fights infection.

As an additional or alternative activity, learners could work in small groups to label an outline of the human body

Activity 7

1. Examples of behaviours or actions that may aid the movement of transient pathogens include:
   - placing raw meat next to cooked meat
   - unprotected sex
   - sneezing without covering the mouth
   - not washing hands properly or frequently
   - not cleaning properly
   - not disinfecting high-risk areas or objects
   - inadequate food storage arrangements, unhygienic food preparation and cooking.

2. Objects that might easily become infected by transient pathogens include towels, dishcloths, cutlery, dirty dressings, hands and fingernails, food particles and any surfaces, especially in sluices, toilets and bathrooms.

Activity 8

1. Root vegetables must be washed thoroughly before eating to remove any soil, which is a source of pathogenic microbes.

2. Some transient pathogens multiply at low temperatures.

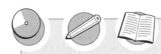

Activity 10

Learners create mind-maps for key terms from the section, writing all the words they can think of associated with each term. This activity could be carried out as a competition in small groups for the most extended or researched answers.

Activity 9

1. Learners state the everyday actions they perform to break the chain of infection. Answers should relate to learners' working practice.

2. Examples of unacceptable practice include:

   - not washing hands between clients
   - not washing hands after going to the toilet or handling waste products
   - changing beds before handling food
   - not wearing protective clothing
   - coming to work when ill.

To reinforce learning about the chain of infection, learners could take part in a dramatisation in which all links in the chain are broken. For example, this could be a role-play in which groups of learners represent each aspect of the chain. The key to the exercise is repetition and discussion of how each group addresses the aspects.

1.3 Understand the essential differences between pathogenic micro-organisms and parasitic organisms, and the diseases they cause

This section lends itself well to learners engaging in research and can be divided into small group tasks, for example:

- Research the description, properties and functions of bacteria, viruses or parasites.

- Research the problem of *Clostridium difficile* and MRSA, specifically in relation to learners' individual job roles.

- Compare diseases caused by bacteria and those caused by viruses, including possible complications.

- Research how HIV originated, or the many outbreaks of influenza.

- Find out about the different types of fungi, yeasts and moulds.

Such research can be suited to any learning style as it gives learners a choice as to how investigate and present their findings. Audio and kinaesthetic learners could create presentations or quizzes, word searches and crosswords. Visual learners could produce posters or displays and examine photos.

Learning about the different parasites is better delivered with photographs of magnified parasites.

Activity 11

Clostridium difficile

- Mrs Maloney should have her own room, en-suite toilet and own toiletries.
- Thorough and regular hand-washing using detergent and an alcohol rub.
- Thorough general cleaning is an effective way of killing spores that may have transferred onto skin or clothes.
- Surfaces such as toilets, bathrooms and bedpans should be cleaned with detergent then disinfected.
- Visitors and staff informed about the need for thorough personal hygiene.
- Keep urinary catheters off the floor and empty bags regularly using disposable gloves.
- Maintain Mrs Maloney's personal hygiene and clean and dry area where catheter enters the body, routinely.

Activity 12

Learners complete the table for the bacterial infections studied in this section (see below) then research at least two other bacterial diseases and add this information to the table.

Disease	Transmission method	Symptoms	Complications
MRSA	By hands (direct contact); may be airborne	High temperature Wounds not healing	Septicaemia
Tuberculosis	Airborne droplets	Coughing sticky sputum	Can infect other organs, e.g. the brain
Legionnaires' disease	Airborne droplets	High temperature	Breathing difficulties, pneumonia
Tetanus	Enters the blood via a cut; usually present in soil	Muscles of the limbs and back tighten	The jaw may lock with problems swallowing and paralysis

Care scenario: MMR immunisation

1. The health visitor might comment that:

   - it is better to protect the child against measles, mumps and rubella than to take the chance that he or she will not catch these diseases

   - the fewer children who are immunised against MMR, the greater the likelihood that these diseases will become prevalent again in the UK

   - there is no recognised medical evidence to support the claim that MMR causes autism.

2. The health visitor should inform parents of the potential complications arising from measles, for example it can cause brain inflammation and brain damage.

Activity 13

Learners complete the table for the viral infections studied in this section (see below) then research at least two other viral diseases and add this information to the table.

Disease	Transmission method	Symptoms	Complications
HIV	Via the blood, semen and vaginal secretions	Weakening of the immune system	Progresses to AIDS; difficulties warding off infections
Measles	Airborne	Fever, runny nose, cough, rash on face and trunk	Can affect the brain
Hepatitis B	Via the blood, semen and vaginal secretions	Fever, nausea, vomiting, liver complaints	Jaundice and anaemia
Mumps	Airborne	Swelling of the glands each side or one side of the jaw	In males can cause infertility
Chickenpox	Airborne and direct contact	Tiny red spots with yellow centres that itch	Brain infection: rare but more severe in older children and adults when shingles can arise
Influenza	Airborne and direct contact	Fever, aching limbs, headaches, gastric problems	Respiratory distress/ pneumonia
Gastro-enteritis	Food and water	Vomiting and diarrhoea	Dehydration

Care scenario: Leila

1. It will be necessary to reassure Leila that thrush is quite common, and is often brought on by taking a course of antibiotics. The treatment is simple and effective and will relieve any itching or soreness.

2. Advice to give Leila about how to prevent a thrush infection includes:

   - be aware of the consequences of taking antibiotics (they can kill the body's normal flora)

   - avoid too much warmth around the groin, for example hot baths and tight clothing

   - avoid sugary foods and alcohol.

Activity 14

Signs of fungal infections are rashes consisting of slightly raised red spots in close proximity or in circles (ringworm). There may also be complaints of itching or soreness in warm damp areas, e.g. beards, groins, armpits.

1.4 Understand how pathogenic micro-organisms grow and spread

The material in this section provides various opportunities for practical applications suited to kinaesthetic and visual learners. For example, pieces of bread, cheese, cake or other foodstuffs (not raw meat) could be placed in sealed dishes and different temperature mediums, e.g. outside or in a warm room. The inside of the container can be made moist or left dry. Learners then monitor the growth of the fungus or mould, noting down descriptions and comparisons, and carrying out research to support this work. (Note: Please risk-assess this activity in case of learners with allergies to certain foodstuffs, and do not allow any contact with contaminated food as there is a risk of inhaled spores.)

Activity 15

The different stages by which transient pathogens succeed in causing infection are:

- multiplying in the right environmental conditions

- finding a route of transmission

- entering a host where they multiply further

- exiting the host to be passed on to other surfaces and hosts.

Care scenario: Mary

1. The risks posed by Mary's actions are cross-contamination from the urine to the food or directly to the second client. Other individuals in the setting who come into contact with Mary, the second client or any of the surfaces or objects Mary or the second client has touched will also be at risk of cross-contamination.

2. Mary should be informed of the dangers of cross-contamination and the need to avoid this by thorough hand-washing after every job and before attending to another task and/or client.

The Reflection activity on page 37 asks learners what they do in their care routines to help people develop a stronger immune system. Encourage them to consider the following:

- a healthy nutritious diet high in protein and vitamin C (fruit and vegetables)
- fresh air and exercise where possible
- sleep and rest
- a positive and peaceful environment with recreational activities easily accessible
- contact with family and friends.

Activity 16

Term	Role in growth and spread of pathogens
Reservoir	Area that contains pathogens and provides the right conditions for their growth. Source of their transmission by direct or indirect contact
Nutrients	Food for pathogenic microbes. Supports their growth and multiplication
Time	The more time in which pathogens are left undisturbed, the greater the number and the greater the risk of infection
Warmth	Ideal temperature range for growth of pathogens is 20–45 degrees Celsius. At these temperatures, most pathogens multiply quickly
Moisture	A slightly moist environment helps pathogens grow and multiply quickly
Oxygen	Most pathogens require oxygen for growth. Anaerobic microbes grow without oxygen

Activity 17

1. Examples of pathogens expelled in a sneeze are *Staphylococcus aureas* (bacteria) and influenza (virus).

2. Conditions that would contribute to a widespread flu epidemic include:

   - crowded conditions, e.g. lots of people gathered together in a cinema or many people living in a household (resulting in a high number of airborne organisms)
   - movement and global travel (people with little resistance coming into contact with 'new' diseases).

To extend this activity, ask learners to research data from when people lived in overcrowded conditions in the UK and compare their findings with today's living conditions. Use an OHP to highlight what happened in the period when children started school, for example in 1870 there were various outbreaks of measles, chickenpox and other communicable diseases.

Care scenario: Lucy

1. Although Lucy sneezes into her handkerchief, it is loosely placed in her long sleeve so may contact other surfaces and contaminate them.

2. Lucy's handkerchief may come into contact with the clean sheet, which could then contact Mrs Andrew's bed sore.

3. The correct procedure Lucy should have followed is:
   - not to come to work until recovered from the cold
   - to use a disposable tissue
   - to wash her hands immediately after sneezing and before continuing the bed change.

4. MRSA infection is common in hospitals and homes because *Staphylococcus aureas* has become resistant to antibiotics (methicillin resistant). MRSA is passed to others when care workers and medical staff do not wash their hands properly.

Activity 18

1. Best-before dates indicate the date after which the quality of the food reduces. Use-by dates are given on more perishable items because there is a high risk of contamination if the food is not consumed by this date.

2. Measures to prevent food poisoning and gastro-enteric infections:
   - hand-washing after toilet use, after handling raw food and before preparing cooked food
   - clean surfaces after use
   - observe use-by dates
   - correct storage of food in low temperatures if cook–chill produce (dairy, eggs, meat, cheese)
   - separate chopping boards
   - cover all food and protect from flies and pests
   - cook sufficiently
   - chill sufficiently.

Care scenario: Listeriosis

1. Soft cheeses, cook–chill produce and pâté are more likely to carry the bacteria *Listeria monocytogenes* because this organism likes low temperatures and can grow in a fridge.

2. Steps to prevent individuals coming into contact with the bacterium include:
   - use-by dates must be strictly adhered to
   - the temperature of the fridge should be checked on every shift for the correct temperature (between 0 and 5 degrees Celsius)
   - ensure that the fridge door is not left open at any time.

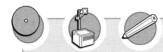

Activity 19

1. *Dust* – clean as you go; keep the area surrounding the individual free from dust.

2. *Flies* – cover all food in the kitchen; install fly screens or electronic 'zappers'.

3. *Blood* – wear protective gloves and clothing; dispose of soiled dressings in clinical waste bags; wash hands thoroughly.

4. *Faeces* – wash hands after disposing of bedpans or attending to soiled beds; wear disposable gloves when collecting specimens.

5. *Urine* – wear protective gloves while in contact with catheter bags or specimens and wash hands thoroughly afterwards; ensure catheter bags are disposed of correctly or emptied using a clinically clean technique.

6. *Nasal mucus/sputum* – if this is being regularly discharged, individuals should have a frequent supply of disposable containers with lids; use disposable gloves to dispose of these.

To extend this activity, learners could create prevention posters or produce their own acetates for a presentation on good practice.

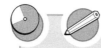

Activity 20

1. False
2. False
3. False
4. True
5. False
6. False
7. True
8. False

Where answers are false, encourage learners to explain why and come up with a 'correct' alternative statement.

2. Preventing and controlling the spread of infection

2.1 Understand the standard precautions to prevent infection and its spread

The aims of this section are to highlight how infections are spread. It should be stressed that the very young, older people, the sick and immuno-suppressed have less resistance to pathogens.

It will be useful to keep reminding learners to reflect on good practice and to challenge any practice they think may be detrimental to individuals. Continual monitoring of the environment is essential, and infection control is everybody's responsibility. It may be helpful to have these two principles in sight at all times, perhaps on a poster, where you can draw attention to it whenever issues arise.

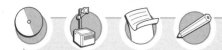
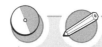

Activity 21

The times and circumstances when a thorough hand-wash should be performed are:

- on arrival at an individual's home or room
- before provision of personal/intimate care
- after performing duties
- after using the toilet
- before preparing food
- before and after bed-making
- after handling waste (kitchen or bodily)
- after removing and disposing of gloves
- on leaving the individual's home or room.

Activity 23

The checklist of hand-washing facilities should include the following:

- clean basins at accessible points and strategically placed
- non-touch taps
- a good supply of liquid soap
- paper towels or hand-dryers
- a supply of sanitiser
- a foot-operated pedal bin.

Activity 22: Aseptic techniques/universal precautions

Learners need to appreciate that catheterisation and aseptic techniques are performed by qualified staff. It is paramount that understanding of the non-touch procedures is of a consistently high standard. Other procedures will include wound dressings, changing three-way taps on Hickman lines (for administration of drugs into veins by qualified staff only), and any procedure that is invasive and involves contact with internal tissues or wounds.

Activity 24

1. You should change into your uniform when you arrive for duty because bacteria may be present on your own clothing. Also, if you change into your uniform at home it may become contaminated before arrival on duty.

2. Jewellery could be a source of contamination and loose parts may contaminate wounds.

3. Wearing goggles prevents splashes of blood or contaminated body fluids entering the eyes during risky procedures. A mask helps to prevent airborne micro-organisms being breathed in or breathed onto others.

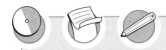

Activity 25

Learners should include the following information when explaining the need to dress appropriately:

- wear a clean uniform daily and change during the shift if it becomes soiled
- soiling may contaminate individuals, food or other objects
- ensure that little make-up is worn as this is a source of contamination
- open-toed shoes are a possible source of contamination so should be avoided
- hair should be worn off the face or tied up
- keep nails short and do not wear nail varnish.

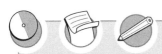

Activity 26

Learners describe how their duties ensure they work from clean areas and tasks to dirty ones. Possible answers include:

- the serving of food prior to dealing with waste disposal
- assisting individuals to wash or bathe prior to handling dirty laundry
- dressing and covering a wound before dusting a room.

Care scenario: Preparation for isolation

1. Provision to be made for Mr Black and care staff:

   - Check the environment for clean wash basins and toilet area; a good supply of paper towels, liquid soap, hand gels, pedal bins; adequate ventilation.
   - Check that Mr Black has his own supply of toiletries, towels and clothing.
   - Place supplies in the room such as dressings, scissors, tape, disposable aprons, gloves, masks, waste skips and clinical waste bags (labelled). Linen should go into red bags.
   - Mr Black to have his own set of cutlery and crockery.
   - Disinfectant to remain in the room.

Activity 27

1. Visitors and medical staff pose a threat to individuals who need isolation nursing.

2. To minimise these risks:

   - inform every visitor verbally of the necessary precautions
   - ensure that a sign reminding visitors and medical staff of the necessary precautions is displayed prominently
   - discourage visitors if a cold or other infection is suspected.

Care scenario: Rubella

1. A second 'booster' rubella vaccination is needed at 4 years to increase the amount of protection when children start school (a vulnerable time).

2. By immunising most people in the UK against rubella the disease will be almost eradicated.

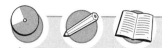

Activity 28

Travel immunisations required:

- Dominican Republic – diphtheria, hepatitis A, hepatitis B, rabies, tetanus, tuberculosis, typhoid.
- India – cholera, hepatitis A, hepatitis B, Japanese B encephalitis, meningococcal meningitis, poliomyelitis, rabies, tetanus, tuberculosis, typhoid, yellow fever.
- Kenya – cholera, hepatitis A, hepatitis B, meningococcal meningitis, rabies, tetanus, tuberculosis, typhoid, yellow fever.

Care scenario: Changing linen

1. The sequence followed and checks made from changing bed linen to collecting lunches on trays and serving to clients in bed is:
   - after placing dirty laundry in bags, wash hands thoroughly
   - check that hot food is indeed hot and cold food chilled
   - check that food is covered
   - enable individual to clean own hands
   - protect bedding and bedclothes.

Care scenario: Safe procedures checklist

1. Learners should complete the chart as follows.

Procedure	What to do	Why it is necessary
Sharps disposal	Put into sharps bin without re-sheathing and check bin is no more than two-thirds full	Re-sheathing is a risk in terms of sustaining a needlestick injury
Handling and serving of food	Wash and dry hands thoroughly; never cough or sneeze over food	Hands carry pathogens that could easily be transmitted to food. Airborne organisms may contaminate food
Management of soiled dressings	Keep separate from clean items; handle using disposable gloves and place in clinical waste bags	To avoid contamination with clean items
Management of soiled laundry	Keep separate from clean items; handle using disposable gloves and place in clinical waste bags	To avoid contamination with clean items

2.2 Understand the correct procedures for handling, storage and disposal of waste

Two of the aims of this section are for learners to become familiar with the different types of waste disposal and know how household waste, clinical waste and biological spillages are dealt with. Learning strategies for this could include:

- *Kinaesthetic and visual learning style* – collect containers for the disposal of clinical waste and display these in a presentation format.
- *Audio learning style* – learners could interview staff about safe disposal techniques.
- *Research* – learners could research the hazards caused by unsafe waste disposal, including biological spillages.

While studying this section, it will be useful to consider relevant current legislation (described in Section 3), particularly the COSHH regulations. Links to practice should also be made. For example, work plans and routines should highlight storage areas for waste and the necessary provisions, such as yellow clinical waste bags.

Activity 29

What to do when a torn yellow bag spills its contents over the floor:

1. Put on disposable gloves.
2. Place a bag over the split bag.
3. Ensure the waste is in its proper designated area.
4. Clean and disinfect the floor area affected.
5. Remove and dispose of gloves and wash hands.

2.3 Understand decontamination techniques

The following research activities can assist learning about decontamination techniques:

- Small groups can research cleaning techniques for low-, medium- and high-risk objects and areas. To present this visually will help all learning styles.

- Learners can research the different ways to disinfect areas and sterilise equipment. They should become familiar with the heat, radiation and chemical processes of disinfection.

- Decontamination techniques could be explored by small groups using products found in the workplace. Comparisons with other brands, for example

comparing the properties on the labels, may help learners understand the difference between cleaning materials and disinfectants.

Activity 30

1. Wooden floor – low risk
2. Surgical scissors – high risk
3. Urinal – high risk
4. Window blind – low risk
5. Shared books – medium risk
6. Toilet seats – high risk
7. Door handles – high risk
8. Food trolleys – medium risk
9. Mattress – medium risk
10. Chopping board for raw meat – high risk

3. Legislation relevant to infection prevention and control

3.1 Understand the legislation, regulations and guidance that govern infection prevention and control

This section guides learners through the legislation they need to understand and commit to when ensuring that their actions minimise infections. The tutor's aim is to highlight this while continually referring to working practice, so learners are clear how the laws impact on their role. The aim should also be to highlight the potential consequences of non-compliance, so learners realise the importance of committing to good practice.

Teaching legislation can be tedious, so it might help to give learners the responsibility of finding out for themselves then presenting their findings to the whole group. Make sure that the focus is on how legislation translates into working practice. You should also discuss the variations in practice according to different types of settings. Learners might also enjoy testing one another, for example using laminated cards. An objective can be to match the requirements to the legislation, which should suit all learning styles.

(Please note that the information given on legislation is accurate at the time of going to print.)

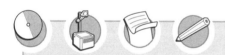

Activity 31

What should appear on labels on medications and cleaning fluids:

- hazard-warning labels – these should be checked for correct instructions of how to use the substance and what not to mix it with.
- expiry dates on medications.
- correct storage instructions, for example medication may need to be stored in a fridge.

Activity 32

Actions to be taken under the Food Safety Act following an outbreak of food poisoning are:

1. Suspect food poisoning and inform manager.
2. Report the signs and symptoms to the environmental health department.
3. Checks must be made to avoid further contamination.

Activity 33

Laws that the settings and care workers have broken:

1. Health and Safety at Work Act (1974)
2. Management of Health and Safety at Work Act (amended 1994)
3. Control of Substances Hazardous to Health (COSHH) Regulations (2002)
4. Reporting of Injuries, Diseases and Dangerous Occurrences Regulations (RIDDOR) (1995)

3.2 Understand the organisation's policies and procedures with regard to infection prevention and control

It is important for learners to appreciate that different care settings will have different policies and procedures regarding infection prevention and control. For example, it is impossible in an individual's private home to implement the procedures of a large organisation such as a hospital. The Look it up activity on page 75 (question 1) asks learners to research the differences in approach for different settings. Conclude this research with a group discussion of their findings.

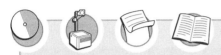

Activity 34

Learners carry out a check of their workplace to identify information and guidance on good hygiene practice. Learners could present their findings using a variety of formats, for example using pictures (with permission from workplace manager), OHP or verbal report.

4. Roles, responsibilities and boundaries

4.1   Understand the roles and responsibilities of personnel in relation to infection prevention and control

Section 4 focuses on a range of professional and non-professional people and their role in minimising infections. The aim is to highlight how everyone must work as a team and communicate concerns, either orally or in writing. Once again, learners will need to reflect on their own working experiences and consider the relevant legislation. Activities in this section are designed to encourage

reflection, particularly on the whereabouts of different people and how infections can 'infiltrate' to environments in care settings.

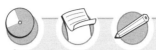

Activity 35

Learners devise an information sheet for new staff to use in their induction period. Ideally this will be in the format of a typical shift and will identify the rooms in which staff will be working. Listing the hazards by area and the actions needed to avoid these is one way to help the new staff member avoid or minimise them. Learners can be encouraged to make sheets interesting by adding their own warning icons (good for visual learners).

Activity 36

1. Tomas should be told about the pathogens he may be spreading by leaving his soiled dressings on the kitchen work surface. These may contaminate other items of food or the work surface, which in turn could contaminate food.
2. Samira's rash may be caused by a parasite such as scabies and may need treatment.
3. Hilda's incontinence pads may harbour pathogens if they linger on her skin for too long, causing nasty sores. The pads must be changed regularly.

When reporting these incidents learners should give both a verbal report to the line manager and a written report. The written report should be signed and dated, documenting the advice given and any actions taken.

Care scenario: Marie

1. The ways in which Marie failed to follow good practice procedures are:
   - she should have taken the laundry skip to the bedside
   - she allowed the bed linen to trail on the floor
   - she should have washed her hands after changing the bed, in between clients, before and after attending to food and after emptying the catheter
   - she did not assist Mrs Kaur to wash her hands before lunch
   - she should have put on disposable gloves before emptying the catheter bag
   - she left a specimen on a table instead of placing this in the specimens fridge.

Care scenario: The gardener and the cook

1. Potential hazards introduced by the gardener and the cook include:
   - leaving raw unwashed vegetables on the kitchen work surface
   - leaving vegetables next to the raw meat (direct contamination)

Activity 37

1. By interviewing initially then supervision and checking and arranging training.
2. In meetings; by distributing memos and ensuring that procedures are prominently displayed.
3. Regular supervision and appraisals; receiving reports from line managers; checking outcomes of training.

4. Isolate the individual and seek medical advice. Brief all staff and provide necessary resources for barrier nursing.
5. Show records of cleaning schedules and data to show improvements; carry out hygiene checks on hands; ensure sanitisers are consistently used and re-ordered. Check areas are consistently clean with waste immediately disposed of. Staff to receive frequent training; ensure catering staff are highly trained (qualification records). Contracted pest control firms to confirm home is pest-free.

Activity 38

Issues of concern and the appropriate plans of action are:

1. *Individual has diarrhoea and vomiting* – report to line manager and isolate individual if possible. Provide staff with disposable gloves and aprons and ensure sufficient hand-washing facilities and sanitiser are available. If possible, collect specimen.
2. *A wound is not healing* – report to manager and note description of wound. Ensure aseptic technique when dressing and keep individual isolated if possible. Document any medication, particularly antibiotics.
3. *Linen is regularly changed* – check whether this is good practice or because of regular soiling.
4. *Mouse droppings are found in the food cupboard* – check pest control contract and cleaning schedules. Also check state of storage. Dispose of any suspect damaged packaging.

- not washing and disinfecting the work surfaces
- not washing hands.

2. What the gardener and the cook *should* have done to maintain control of infection:
   - leave the vegetables in a suitable container away from surfaces where food will be prepared
   - when the cook saw the unwashed vegetables she should have moved them straight away and washed and disinfected the work surfaces, then washed her hands
- the cook should inform the gardener not to leave unwashed vegetables on the work surface.

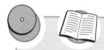

Activity 39

Learners carry out research into the role of the different organisations and teams listed. This activity could be conducted in pairs or small groups, with each pair/group responsible for finding out about one of the organisations/teams listed. Pairs and groups can then swap to compare findings or a class discussion could be held.

4.2 Understand the roles and responsibilities of the worker with regard to following the organisation's policies and procedures

For the Look it up activity on page 84 and the Reflection activity on page 87, learners are asked about how certain information is recorded in their setting.

When documenting the care of individuals, specific guidance will depend on the environment in which the learner works. However, there should be commonality in terms of the information recorded on an accident report form (what happened; the name and age of the victim; the outcome was; treatment given; medical history; dates, times and two signatures).

Learners are then asked to use the knowledge gained in this section to anticipate what food management documentation will record (Reflection activity page 88). Answers can be related to a HACCP point as follows:

- identify the risks in preparing, cooking and serving food
- analyse the hazards involved
- plan to avoid the hazards, for example cook to a sufficiently high temperature
- monitor and evaluate safety measures.

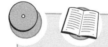

Activity 40

Learners complete the table by assessing their own organisation against the criteria for auditing high standards of infection control. If they have ticked the 'No' column, the appropriate actions are described below.

1. Report to line manager; ensure supplies are available as soon as possible.
2. Arrange for updates of qualified staff and for new staff to have induction information on infection control.
3. Instigate practical sessions for training procedures. Check that staff know how to wash hands properly, wear protective clothing and dispose of sharps safely.

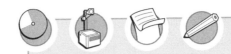

Care scenario: Amelia

Correct procedure:

- explain to Amelia the need for the specimen
- label the appropriate container and include date and time
- once the sample has been transferred from the bedpan, place the container in a sealed bag using disposable gloves
- dispose of the gloves and wash hands thoroughly
- attach the request from the doctor
- check that the reason for the sample has been recorded.

Care scenario: Advising the visitor

Explain politely the need for all visitors to adhere to infection control measures. Explain that the hospital or setting exercises these controls to minimise infection and for the well-being of all individuals. Ask the visitor to wash his hands. (Learners should note that hand-washing is best done *before*

Activity 41

Learners complete the flow chart to identify what else needs to be assessed when identifying hazards in the workplace. This activity is best carried out in small groups. Feedback and discussion should address different types of care settings. Possible answers include:

- *Domiciliary care*: kitchen area; clean surfaces; clean utensils; clean cloths; foods covered.
- *Care home*: warm well-ventilated room; clean bedding; space around the bed area; clean clothes daily; washing facilities close by; provision of disposable supplies.
- *Hospital isolation*: disposable equipment and resources; PPE; red bags for soiled linen.

visitors go into the room where friends and relatives are.)

Activity 42

Hazard	Risk
1. Beds positioned too close together	Cross-contamination via airborne pathogens
2. Communal toilet	Cross-contamination arising from frequent use by ill and weak individuals
3. Peeling paint	Provides a reservoir in which pathogens multiply
4. Windows closed	Stale air increases the risk of airborne pathogens
5. Open bins next to beds	Provides a reservoir in which pathogens multiply; risk of cross-contamination to ill or weak individuals

4.3 Understand the need to carry out risk assessments when dealing with individuals and potentially contaminated materials

Care scenario: Keeping good records

1. To show good hygiene and food-safety practice, the chef will need to prove that he keeps records of due diligence. These include pest control contracts, cleaning schedules, use of reputable suppliers for food purchase and training records of staff. He will also need to show that procedures are well implemented.

For the Reflection activity on page 98, learners are asked to state how they would know if measures to minimise infection were working. Elicit from them the following responses:

- the infection rate is reduced
- the environment is clean
- lab results are clear
- staff remain vigilant at all times.

Student log

The following tables have been reproduced with the kind permission of Skills for Care. Use these tables to log your progress during your training and record the learning outcomes you have covered. The tables may also be used to map the content of an NVQ qualification or other relevant training course. For full details of how the knowledge set for dementia cross-references NVQ units, Common Induction Standards and GSCC Code of Practice (workers), please see the Skills for Care knowledge set document. A link to the documents on the skillsforcare.org.uk website has been made available at www.heinemann.co.uk/hotlinks. Simply enter the express code 2307P when you access the site.

Main area	Learning outcome	Learning outcome achieved (manager's or trainer's signature)	Date
1. Cause and spread of infection	1.1 Understand the definition of infection and colonisation: ■ Systemic infection (affects the whole body) ■ Localised infection (confined to a specific area) ■ Difference between infection and colonisation		
	1.2 Understand how micro-organisms cause infection: ■ Normal flora (usually non-pathogenic micro-organisms that are mostly helpful within the body) ■ Transient flora (often pathogenic micro-organisms that are harmful, disease-causing) ■ The chain of infection		
	1.3 Understand the essential differences between pathogenic micro-organisms and parasitic organisms, and the diseases they cause: ■ Bacteria, e.g. MRSA, tuberculosis, legionnaires' disease, tetanus ■ Viruses, e.g. HIV, Hepatitis B, measles, mumps, cold/influenza, viral gastro-enteritis ■ Fungi, e.g. thrush, athlete's foot, ringworm ■ Parasites, e.g. scabies, lice		

Main area	Learning outcome	Learning outcome achieved (manager's or trainer's signature)	Date
	1.4 Understand how pathogenic micro-organisms grow and spread: • Growth (reservoir, food, moisture, warmth, time) • Spread (contact, droplet, flies, fingers, fomites, faeces, air dust, water, food)		
2. Preventing and controlling the spread of infection	2.1 Understand the standard precautions to prevent infection and its spread: • Hand hygiene: correct hand washing technique, use of alcohol gels and other antiseptics, hand drying, skin care, facilities required • Use of appropriate personal protective equipment (PPE) • General cleanliness (personal, environmental, materials, equipment) • Principles of isolation nursing • General cleanliness (personal, environmental, equipment, materials) • Immunisation (occupational health for staff, general public and individuals) • Following correct/safe practice procedures • Prevention of sharps injury • Management of outbreaks of infection • Food handling • Soiled laundry management		

Main area	Learning outcome	Learning outcome achieved (manager's or trainer's signature)	Date
	2.2 Understand the correct procedures for handling, storage and disposal of waste (using the correct colour-coded bag or bin): ■ Sharps ■ Household waste ■ Clinical/hazardous waste ■ Biological spillages		
	2.3 Understand decontamination techniques: ■ Low risk (e.g. floors, furniture, mobility aids) ■ Medium risk (e.g. bedpans, urinals, commodes) ■ High risk (e.g. instruments used for invasive techniques) **NB Each item requires assessing for cleaning, disinfection or sterilisation to be carried out in line with policy. Always seek advice following their use on individuals with infection.**		
3. Legislation relevant to infection prevention and control	3.1 Understand the legislation, regulations and guidance that govern infection prevention and control: ■ Health and Safety at work Act 1974 ■ Management of Health and Safety at Work Act (amended 1994) ■ The Public Health (Control of Diseases) Act 1984 ■ Food Safety Act 1990 ■ COSHH 2002 ■ RIDDOR 1995 ■ The Public Health (Infectious Diseases) Regulation 1988		

Main area	Learning outcome	Learning outcome achieved (manager's or trainer's signature)	Date
	■ The Food Safety (General Food Hygiene) Regulation (Department of Health 1995) ■ The Environmental Protection *(Duty of Care)* Regulations (1991) ■ Health Protection Agency Bill ■ Hazardous Waste Regulations 2005 ■ NICE (National Institute for Clinical Excellence) Guideline 2 June 2003 **NB This list of legislation, regulations and guidance is given as an example and is subject to change. It is important when designing learning packages, in-house training, etc. that the most recent legislation, regulations and guidance are included and that the learning relates to the role of the worker.**		
	3.2 Understand the organisation's policies and procedures with regard to infection prevention and control		
4. Roles, respon-sibilities and boun-daries	4.1 Understand the roles and responsibilities of personnel in relation to infection prevention and control: ■ Care worker ■ Non-care workers (gardeners, cooks, drivers, administrators, etc) ■ Manager ■ The organisation ■ Specialist personnel (infection control nurses and doctors, Environmental Health Officer, Health Protection Units)		

Main area	Learning outcome	Learning outcome achieved (manager's or trainer's signature)	Date
	4.2 Understand the roles and responsibilities of the worker with regard to following the organisation's policies and procedures: ■ Reporting of infectious or notifiable diseases and outbreaks ■ Seeking advice and guidance ■ Admissions, transfers and discharges of individuals ■ Documentation and record keeping in relation to infection ■ Following the death of a individual ■ Handling, collection and storing of specimens (urine (MSU/CSU), faeces, blood, vomit, sputum, wound swabs) ■ Encourage all visitors to comply with hygiene policies and procedures		
	4.3 Understand the need to carry out risk assessment when dealing with individuals and potentially contaminated materials: ■ Identify the hazard(s) ■ Assess the risk ■ Record the risk ■ Remove/reduce the risk ■ Review the risk regularly		

Websites

Page 71   Look it up: How does the work of the Health Protection Agency affect your work in the healthcare sector? Website address: www.hpa.org.uk

Page 72   Look it up: Visit the National Institute for Health and Clinical Excellence (NICE) website to find out more about the range of informative publications on preventing infection in care settings.
Guidance available at www.nice.org.uk/guidance/CG2#documents

Page 74   Look it up: The Royal College of Nursing has created an infection control checklist as part of its 'Wipe it Out' campaign to combat MRSA. http://www.rcn.org.uk/resources/mrsa/downloads/Wipe_it_out-Good_practice_in_infection_prevention_and_control.pdf (Appendix 1)

Page 85   Look it up: Access examples of websites on good practice in relation to infection control:
- www.rcn.org.uk (Royal College of Nursing)
- www.nice.org.uk (National Institute for Health and Clinical Excellence)
- www.nhs.uk (NHS in England)
- www.healthline.com (Healthline – a medically guided search engine); www.mulho.com (Mulberry House – one of the UK's main care training and consultancy providers)
- www.skillsforcare.com (Skills for Care – provides resources, information and advice to support the development of the adult social care workforces in England)
- www.doh.gov.uk (Department of Health)

Page 87   The National Institute for Health and Clinical Excellence (NICE) has provided leaflets to help individuals with admissions, transfers and discharges which are free of charge. You will be able to order copies of these via their website (www.nice.org.uk).

Glossary

antigen   substance which the body recognises as unknown and sets out to destroy

audit   a checking process to ensure standards are maintained

binary fission   process by which a single-celled organism splits into two cells of roughly equal size

carrier   a person infected with a pathogen which remains in the body but causes no signs of illness

colonisation   when a microbe establishes itself in a particular environment such as a body surface, although does not necessarily produce disease

contagious   infection easily spread from one person to another

contamination   when something has become infected or polluted

cross-infection   process by which micro-organisms on one object or person transfer to another object or person (e.g. dishcloth to food)

decontamination   to make free from contaminants

DNA and RNA   deoxyribonucleic acid are proteins that provide the genetic blueprint for the physical characteristics of all living organisms

epidemic   widespread outbreak of disease that affects many people at one time

excrete   to get rid of waste from the body

fomite   an item or piece of equipment, for example towels, face cloths, tables, chairs, books, toys, that can pass on a disease from an infected person to others

immunity   the body's ability to ward off infection. This can be natural, as in the case of antibodies fighting antigens, or artificial, for example the result of immunisation or vaccination

incubation   the time taken for a pathogen or its toxins to cause the signs and symptoms of disease

infection   the presence of microbes in the body which cause illness

inflammatory response   a response whereby white cell activity and antibodies at the site of infection have caused redness, swelling and the collection of pus (dead white cells)

inoculation   injecting a vaccine (made artificially) to protect the body against pathogens which cause disease. The terms 'inoculation' and 'immunisation' are often used interchangeably

Knowledge set for infection prevention and control

isolation   a method of physical protection by caring for an individual (who has a specific infection requiring this type of care) in a single room

last offices   the final care duty carried out for a person who has died. It involves bathing the person and dressing him or her in a clean gown

localised infection   infection affecting a specific area of the body, for example a finger or knee

metabolism   the process by which cells gain energy from food and turn out waste products

microbe   micro-organism

mortuary   place where dead bodies are kept before burial or cremation

normal floras   helpful non-pathogenic organisms

notifiable disease   disease that must be reported to the appropriate authorities. Examples of notifiable diseases are those that may cause epidemic or pandemic outbreaks, including smallpox, anthrax and chickenpox

pandemic   epidemic over a wide area, i.e. outbreak of disease affecting people in many different countries at the same time

pathogen   micro-organism with the ability to cause disease

pH   percentage of hydrogen ions. The pH scale ranges from 0 (strongly acidic) to 14.0 (strongly alkaline), with 7.0 as neutral (neither acidic or alkaline)

portal of entry   how a pathogen enters the body

portal of exit   how a pathogen leaves the body

precautions   safety measures to protect against possible danger, illness or injury

reservoir   area which contains pathogenic micro-organisms and provides the right conditions for their growth

responsible organism   pathogenic micro-organism that causes disease

secretion   substance produced by the cells of the body, for example tears or mucus

sign   what you can see about a person when he or she is unwell

spores   protective coatings on some bacteria that make them hard to destory even at very high or low temperatures. If conditions become favourable, the spores germinate to enable the bacteria to multiply

symptom   what a person may complain of when he or she is unwell, for example feeling sick

systemic infection   infection affecting the whole body

toxins   poisons released from pathogenic microbes

transient floras   organisms easily acquired on the hands through touch and transferable to another person or surface

transmission   the passing on of a disease-causing organism

Index

Knowledge Sets

Take a look at more titles in the Knowledge Sets series...

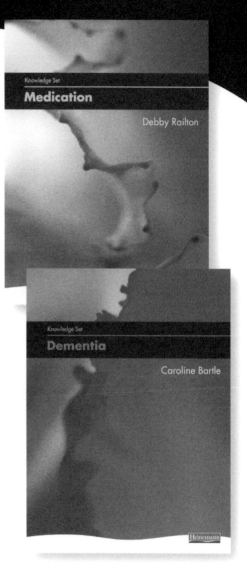

- ◆ Practical handbooks covering dementia and medication for workers, managers and trainers in adult social care.

- ◆ Information delivered in easy-to-manage chunks to make the learning process quick and simple.

- ◆ Content organised around learning outcomes to help care workers get the most out of their learning.

- ◆ Each book enables workers to record their training experience and helps trainers and managers prove they are delivering consistent training.

Knowledge Set for Dementia
978 0 435402 30 3

Knowledge Set for Medication
978 0 435402 31 0

Visit your local bookshop, go to www.harcourt.co.uk/care, or contact our Customer Services team on 01865 888118 for further information.

Sign up for the FREE health and social care eNewsletter at www.harcourt.co.uk/vocnews.